Nutritional Diseases

Douglas A. Eagles

NUTRITIONAL DISEASES

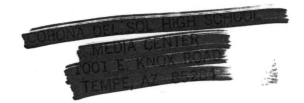

FRANKLIN WATTS
NEW YORK|LONDON|TORONTO|SYDNEY|1987
A FIRST BOOK

Photographs courtesy of Photo Researchers, Inc.:
pp. 18 (Leonard Lee Rue II), 4 (Susan Rosenberg),
80 (Wasyl Szkodzinsky); H. Armstrong Roberts: p. 25;
Taurus Photos: pp. 26 (Science Photo Library), 49 .
(David M. Phillips), 54 (Martin M. Rotker); WHO Photo:
p. 33 (J.P. Assal); L.V. Bergman and Associates, Inc.:

Library of Congress Cataloging in Publication Data

Eagles, Douglas A.
  Nutritional diseases.

  (A First book)
  Bibliography: p.
  Includes index.
  Summary: Explains the development, symptoms,
treatment, and possible prevention of such diseases as
osteoporosis, arteriosclerosis, phenylketonuria, and
diabetes, as well as conditions such as anorexia
and bulemia, which are the result of inadequate nutrition.
  1. Nutrition disorders—Juvenile literature.
2. Nutritionally induced diseases—Juvenile
literature. [1. Nutritionally induced diseases.
2. Eating disorders] I. Title.
RC620.E18 1987   616.3'9   87-8124
ISBN 0-531-10391-9

Contents

Nutritional Diseases

Chapter One

PHYSIOLOGY
AND BIOCHEMISTRY

Eating is so basic and natural that most people rarely think much about it, though we are all aware that eating is essential for survival. Eating well is also essential for good health and, for people who are still growing, for normal development. In this book we shall consider various aspects of nutrition and of the diseases that result from inadequate nutrition. Before we begin, however, it may be helpful to outline some of the basic facts that are important in understanding how our bodies use the food we eat.

We eat to obtain two things: materials and energy. Some of what we eat eventually becomes a part of our bodies, and some is converted to energy. Some of that energy is used to make parts of our body, to maintain those parts we already have, and to exchange materials in parts of the body with the materials in the food we eat. The rest of the energy is either stored in one of several forms or is used for activity (movement). How our bodies do all of these things is rather complex and is the subject of this book, although we cannot consider all the details. For now, we shall explore some of the basic facts that we need to know in understanding nutrition and nutritional diseases.

(9)

A BIT OF
BIOCHEMISTRY

Biochemistry deals with the chemicals that are important to living organisms and with their reactions with each other. There are many different kinds of chemicals that we must obtain from our food.

By volume or weight, most of the food we eat is of three types: carbohydrates (sugars and starches), fats, and proteins. Carbohydrates and fats are both made from three chemical elements: carbon, hydrogen, and oxygen. When we use their carbohydrates or fats, energy is transferred from them to a molecule called *ATP* (adenosine triphosphate). The materials in the carbohydrates or fats combine with oxygen from the air we breathe and are broken down into two simple molecules: water (H_2O) and carbon dioxide (CO_2). The water is made available to the body just as it is when we drink it, and the carbon dioxide is lost from the body in the air we exhale. (Green plants use the carbon dioxide to make new molecules of carbohydrate.). ATP serves as a sort of all-purpose substance for the short-term storage and transfer of energy.

Proteins are made from five kinds of chemical elements: carbon, hydrogen, oxygen, nitrogen, and sulfur. These elements combine in various ways to make molecules called *amino acids*. There are about twenty different kinds of amino acids. Proteins are made by linking together various combinations of these amino acids. A protein molecule may be quite large, and chains of amino acids may be folded in various ways to produce a complex structure. As we shall see, this structure is very important to the proper functioning of a protein molecule. Proteins may also be used as sources of energy. When we use proteins (obtained from meats and some plants) for energy, carbon dioxide, water, and ATP are produced; in addition, a chemical called *urea* is produced. The body gets rid of the nitrogen that is present in proteins by producing urea (which contains nitrogen) and eliminating it from the body in the urine.

For all three types of food molecules—carbohydrates, fats, and proteins—the amount of energy present is described by the number of calories it is said to contain. A *calorie* is the amount of heat required to warm one gram of water by one degree centigrade. One thousand calories gives a unit called a *kilocalorie*, the amount of heat required to warm one thousand grams of water by one degree centigrade. The "calories" used to measure the amount of energy in foods are really kilocalories.

From here on in this book, when we write "Calories" we really mean kilocalories; the capital C will serve as a reminder.

It may help you remember this to think of the heat that would be produced if the food were burned. Our bodies obtain about the same amount of energy from the food as would be obtained by burning it, except that they obtain this energy at a much lower temperature by a process known as *metabolism*.

To review, the energy obtained by metabolizing fats, carbohydrates, or proteins is first used to make ATP. ATP can be used to do many different kinds of work in the body. For example, ATP is used to provide the energy when a muscle contracts. It also provides the energy that is needed to build new molecules in many different kinds of chemical reactions, including those important for growth.

One important thing that proteins do is serve as *enzymes*. Enzymes are a type of catalyst; that is, they speed up the rates of chemical reactions. Without enzymes, many of the important chemical reactions in the body would not occur at rates fast enough to support living cells and tissues.

Besides carbohydrates, fats, and proteins, there are many other types of chemicals that are required for the body to function properly. Most of them do not provide energy and are required only in very small amounts. For example, it is absolutely essential for good health that we obtain certain vitamins. But our bodies require them only in very small amounts. They are not used as fuel, as the fats, carbohydrates, and—sometimes—proteins may be. Some vitamins are synthesized by the body, and some must be obtained from foods. The lack of any one of them produces characteristic symptoms or diseases, but it is not always clear how the presence of a vitamin prevents the appearance of those symptoms. Some vitamins, such as the B vitamins, act as cofactors, or helpers, for certain enzymes.

The rate at which chemical reactions occur depends on the conditions present. Thus, it is important that many different conditions be maintained in order for our bodies to operate properly. The raw materials needed to make the chemicals our bodies require must be obtained from the diet, and we must have adequate water to serve as a solvent so that all the compounds can be dissolved and made available to react. The rates of chemical reactions are also very dependent on temperature and on pH (a measure of acidity); these variables, too, must be controlled.

A BIT OF PHYSIOLOGY

Physiology is the study of function. Much of physiological research studies how the body regulates its activities so that its internal environment is kept within the narrow limits required by our biochemistry, and how the body adapts to meet the demands imposed upon it. When we are physically active, for example, the body expends great amounts of energy. The immediate source of this energy is ATP in the muscles. Those stores are quickly depleted, however, and the muscles then turn to other molecules containing phosphate (the P in ATP) for short-term replenishment of the ATP. When the demand for energy continues, a sugar—glucose—is used as a source of energy. Whether or not glucose is used to provide energy depends on whether there is enough oxygen available to the muscles. When activity begins and as it continues, the brain receives signals that cause it, in turn, to send signals to the body that cause an increase in the breathing and heart rates. These help to ensure that oxygen is available. If activity continues long enough, starches in the liver and in fats located throughout the body may be used to provide the energy required. The energy required to drive all the chemical reactions in the body ultimately depends upon the use of oxygen. Metabolism involves the energy demands of all of these reactions, and in general the rate of metabolism can be measured as the rate of oxygen use.

The body has many mechanisms available to it for changing its activities. It can increase or decrease the total level of metabolism, and it can control the rates of various reactions with amazing precision. Of course, the brain controls movement and behavior, but it also controls such things as blood pressure. In addition, there is a system of glands, called the *endocrine glands*, that release hormones into the blood. These hormones are carried by the blood to all parts of the body. Tissues and organs react differently to the various hormones released by these glands and may produce their own hormones that in turn act upon still other tissues and organs; thus, the endocrine glands play an important role in regulating bodily function. Together, the brain and endocrine glands control such important functions as heat balance and temperature regulation, eating and water balance, and the transfer of materials among the liver, fat cells, muscles, brain, the digestive system, and other parts of the body. The heart and circulatory system play an important role in such transfers, and they are also under the control of the brain and endocrines.

Under a wide variety of conditions, the body operates in a coordinated way so that all vital functions may be maintained.

Since the energy and materials required for all these activities are obtained from the foods we eat, it is important that the diet be adequate in both the amounts and the types of nutrients that our bodies require. In the chapters that follow, we shall explore the nature of a balanced diet and a few of the many diseases that can result either from an inadequate diet or from an inadequate ability to use a diet that is normally adequate.

Chapter Two

STARVATION

For most of us, the exclamation "Oh, I'm starved!" suggests that we have gone without eating for as long as six or eight hours. Few of us go to bed hungry very often, if at all, and very few of us have gone without eating for more than a day. But those who have gone without eating for a day or so do not find it to be a very difficult or uncomfortable experience; they find that the early "hunger pangs" pass quickly.

This suggests that the body manages quite well without food—at least for short periods. Does the body remain healthy without food available to it? How do our bodies function without food? How long can a person go without eating? In this chapter we will explore these questions and other aspects of this simple, if potentially fatal, change in nutrition.

Let us begin with some terminology. Total starvation, or *marasmus*, is the complete absence of food. Partial starvation includes two other conditions: *undernutrition* and *malnutrition*. *Undernutrition* means that there is not enough food, while *malnutrition* means that some food is available but not enough of the right kinds of food. All of our discussion will assume that adequate water is available.

How long could a person live without eating? Most adults would easily survive for the biblical forty days and forty nights, and some obese people have lived for as long as nine months in near-total starvation! These people resumed eating not when they were about to die but rather when they had finally reached average body weight for their size. Obviously, a person's survival time is increased if there is a large store of body fat, since fat serves as a concentrated store of energy. What other factors determine how long a person might live without eating?

We may liken the body to a reservoir of energy, or a fuel tank. The amount of time the fuel will last depends on how much there is and how rapidly it is used. Recall from chapter one that the term *metabolism* is used to denote all the chemical reactions occurring in the body. Some of these reactions involve breaking down molecules, and others involve building them up. Under normal conditions—that is, when food is present and body weight stays constant—these reactions are in balance. But during growth, there is an excess of the reactions involved in building up body tissues, while during starvation there is an excess of the reactions involved in breaking down body tissues. When children suffer starvation, growth stops.

In general during conditions of starvation, anything that increases the metabolic rate will also decrease survival time. Conditions that affect the rate of metabolism, therefore, also directly affect survival time. Humans and other so-called warm-blooded animals use large amounts of energy obtained from their food to keep their body temperatures fairly constant. When the air temperature falls below a certain level, the only way they can keep warm is to increase the amount of heat they produce. Colder air temperatures, therefore, result in an increased metabolic rate and a shorter survival time. Starving people tend to be unusually sensitive to cold and to dress warmly if they can. Similarly, energy is used in performing physical exercise. As you might expect, starving people tend to be inactive.

There are differences in metabolism between males and females as well; males tend to have higher metabolic rates, though they are also larger and therefore have larger reserves. Women, however, tend to have more fat for their size than do men.

Age also affects the metabolic rate. From infancy to adolescence, the total metabolic rate increases because of the increase in size. It increases even more during puberty, mostly because at this time people experience a rapid increase in growth; then it very slowly declines throughout the rest of our lives. Infants and young children have low total rates of metabolism, but their rates are higher for their size than they are for adults. Because they have small stores of energy in their bodies, they often have short survival times when food is unavailable.

In addition, the state of a person's general health is also an important consideration. For example, a person who has a fever has a high body temperature. This high body temperature is produced by a high rate of metabolism, which tends to shorten survival time. As we shall see later, the types of foods that are available can also affect survival time.

Some useful lessons can be learned from studying the responses of other animals to food shortages. The smallest warm-blooded animals of all are the shrews; they look like small mice. Their diet consists mostly of insects and hummingbirds, which in turn eat plant products such as nectar. Shrews may weigh as little as two or three grams (one-tenth of an ounce). They may starve to death in six hours if they are unable to eat. Hummingbirds can survive longer than this, since they can go through a night without eating. One reason for this is that they can lower their body temperature by as much as ten degrees Centigrade during the night. This occurs due to a reduction in their metabolic rate; its effect is to extend their energy reserves.

Some animals, such as groundhogs (woodchucks), spend most of the winter season without eating, curled up in burrows deep in hibernation. Groundhogs prepare for winter by storing excess body fat during the fall season. (If there is a sudden, severe food shortage, they may enter hibernation at almost any time of the year.) This serves to extend their survival time by making it possible for them to survive without eating until conditions become more favorable—that is, until spring arrives.

So-called cold-blooded animals, such as frogs, turtles, and lizards, do not expand metabolic energy to keep their bodies warmer or cooler than their surroundings. This imposes a different set of problems for these animals, but it gives them greatly extended survival times when food is scarce.

Animals differ in details, but the general patterns of weight loss and change in body composition for all animals are similar during starvation or prolonged periods of fasting. Since our own bodies are of most interest to us, we will focus our attention on humans and on animals very similar to us. Let's first consider the matter of weight loss. Weight loss is usually evaluated in terms of two categories: *sensible* and *insensible* losses. The term *sensible* refers to weight loss that we are aware of or can "sense."

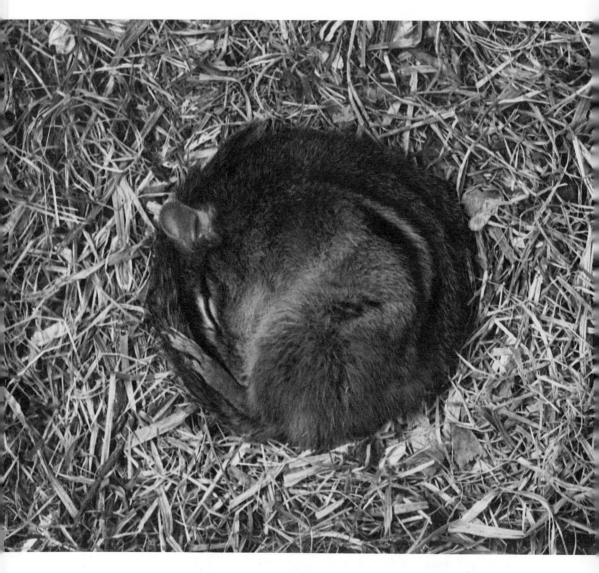

Hibernating animals, such as this chipmunk, are able to store excess body fat during the fall to carry them through the winter months when food is scarce.

Sensible weight losses via the production of urine and feces occur when fasting begins; the rate of weight loss is very high. But once the digestive tract has been emptied, there normally will be no further sensible loss of weight. Urinary losses will continue at a rate that depends on the metabolic rate, though usually they will become quite small, since starving persons tend to become fairly inactive.

After the initial period of sensible weight loss, further losses occur primarily via the insensible route. Weight is lost insensibly—without our awareness of it—through loss of water vapor from the lungs (this can be quite a large factor) and from the skin (usually a small quantity). The rate of these losses depends on the humidity in the air and body temperature. The losses may be considered temporary, since they will be made up by drinking if water is available. A more lasting insensible weight loss occurs due to the loss of carbon dioxide with each breath the person exhales. This carbon dioxide, as well as the nitrogen lost in the urine, comes from the breakdown of body tissues for energy.

You might ask, "When a person loses weight, just where does all the fat (and, perhaps, muscle) go?" The answer is that the fats and carbohydrates that are stored in our bodies eventually are broken down into water and carbon dioxide, as is much of the protein; the remainder of the protein is broken down into various molecules containing nitrogen. The losses of these chemicals—water, carbon dioxide, and nitrogen—represent the loss of materials from the body. Most of our weight is lost this way.

As weight is lost and the body becomes smaller, it requires less energy. Consequently, the metabolic rate slows. Therefore, the rate of weight loss decreases steadily as starvation continues. In addition, as starvation becomes more advanced, the individual becomes less and less active, which also reduces the metabolic rate and the rate of weight loss.

When weight is lost, it is not lost at an equal rate by each of the organs of the body. Table 1 shows the relative losses suffered by different parts of the body during starvation.

When our food supply is unlimited, our bodies use fats, carbohydrates, and proteins in various proportions all the time. But when food is suddenly unavailable, a predictable pattern develops. A person usually utilizes the main blood sugar, glucose, within about twelve hours of the time the fast begins. During those twelve hours, less and less of the energy being used comes from the variety of products resulting from

Table 1

Body Part	Percent Weight Loss at Death
Fat	97
Spleen	69
Pancreas	17
Liver	54
Heart	3
Skeletal muscle	31
Intestine	18
Skin and hair	21
Lungs	18
Brain	3

the breakdown of the last meal. Circulating glucose is utilized rather rapidly by the brain, which uses about two-thirds of the supply, and by the skeletal muscles, which together use about one-third of the supply available. Because the use is rapid, glucose must be produced and released into the blood from some source. At first, most of the glucose comes from the breakdown of a starch, glycogen, in the liver. Later on, about half of the glucose that is produced comes from the kidney. A small amount of glucose also comes from other tissues in the body.

In order to maintain this glucose production, the body requires *enzymes*. Enzymes are catalysts that speed up the rates of other chemical reactions without themselves being used in those reactions. Most enzymes consist largely of protein. Since no protein is being eaten, where does the protein come from during starvation? It comes from proteins already in the body, mainly from proteins in the skeletal muscles. From the first day of the fast, some body protein is being broken down and used. Later in the fast, considerably more protein will be consumed, not for enzyme production but as a last source of energy. In between, after the immediate sources of blood glucose are used up and after some of the liver glycogen has been used up, fat, stored in specialized fat cells, will serve as the main energy reserve.

Two hormones, *insulin* and *glucagon*, play especially important roles in regulating the amount of glucose in the blood and in the directions in which it is transported. Both are secreted by the *pancreas*, a small gland near the stomach. Insulin causes many kinds of cells to absorb glucose from the blood. Fat cells and muscle cells are especially sensitive to this action of insulin. (The brain, incidentally, always takes up glucose very rapidly, and so insulin does not normally have an important effect upon the brain.) This action by insulin is important because it aids in distributing glucose where it is needed for energy production.

Glucose is commonly, but not exclusively, produced in the liver and is then released to the blood. Insulin helps ensure that the muscles, which are very active and require a large energy supply, receive adequate glucose. Insulin also promotes the uptake of glucose by fat cells and ensures that the level of blood sugar will not remain high for long periods of time.

Glucagon has the opposite effect on the blood sugar level. It raises the blood sugar level by promoting the secretion of glucose from the liver, and from other tissues to a lesser extent, into the blood. In a healthy individual, these hormones are secreted together and in balance, jointly regulating the blood glucose and keeping it within a narrow range.

During starvation, the proportions of insulin and glucagon that are secreted change so that relatively less insulin and relatively more glucagon are secreted. This change promotes the loss of glucose from most of the tissues in the body except the brain. It also promotes the breakdown of fat in the fat cells. The fat does not break down into glucose directly but rather is broken down into substances called *fatty acids* and *triglycerides*. These are further changed in the liver and are often converted to glucose. In this way, the body adjusts to the condition of starvation, using its own resources to maintain nearly normal functional conditions. The body actually appears to be well adapted to tolerate starvation. Unless it is extreme, starvation does not lead to serious immediate health problems for normally healthy individuals. Interestingly, some of the oldest people alive today recall frequent periods of hunger as children.

Chapter Three

PROTEIN DEFICIENCY

Good health requires a diet that provides certain essential materials. We need some of them only in rather small amounts. Iron, for example, is necessary because it is an important part of our blood; iodine is important for the proper functioning of the thyroid gland, which in turn affects the rate at which we use our food.

Although many people in the world are starving, many more are suffering from malnutrition due to a lack of adequate protein in their diets. Part of the explanation for this is provided by looking at some very fundamental principles of biology.

First, all our energy comes from the sun. As animals we can warm ourselves in the sun, but beyond that we cannot use the energy from sunlight. We have to obtain it from green plants. Green plants are green because they contain chlorophyll (a pigment that is closely related to the pigment that makes our blood red, hemoglobin. Hemoglobin permits the blood to capture and transport oxygen.) Chlorophyll permits plant tissues to capture light energy and to use that energy to bring carbon dioxide and water together to form glucose. Some of the glucose produced by plants remains glucose, but some of it is changed to starch, and some is changed to cellulose, the woody substance of which most green plants are made.

All animals depend on plants for their food. Some, like cows and sheep and people, eat the plants themselves. Some, like dogs and cats and people, eat the animals that eat the plants. By weight, more than 99 percent of all living things on earth are green plants. Because plants are more abundant than animals, people are more likely to find plants to eat than animals. People in many of the poorer parts of the world are almost exclusively vegetarians, eating very little meat. (Some people also choose to be vegetarians, although many of these people include animal products—milk and eggs—in their diets.) Plants provide adequate energy, and so you might think that this would cause no problems. Unfortunately, many plants contain relatively small quantities of proteins, and these are incomplete; they lack some of the amino acids that people require in their diets.

As we saw in chapter one, proteins play an important role in the structure of the body and an even more important role as enzymes. Each protein is made up of many amino acids. Our bodies can make about fourteen of the twenty kinds of amino acids, but the other six must be provided by the diet. These six are the *essential* amino acids. Without them, enzymes cannot be made. Without enzymes, some chemical reactions in the body cannot occur rapidly enough to meet the body's needs.

In chapter two we considered the body's response to total starvation. The body responds similarly to malnutrition, or to any condition in which there is a reasonably well-balanced diet but too little of everything to meet the body's needs. The activity of the liver, which is important in converting chemicals from one form to another, remains normal. The concentrations and types of proteins in the blood also remain normal.

One reason why many aspects of bodily function remain normal in malnutrition is that some parts of the body are used as reservoirs for substances that are needed. For example, in total starvation the muscles serve as a source of the essential amino acids that were taken in when food was available. Of course, the supply available from the muscles will gradually be exhausted, but until that time the chemistry of the body remains fairly constant. Likewise, when there is simply not enough food, our bodies rely on their own resources to make up the difference.

For people in many parts of the world, plant foods are often available in sufficient quantities to meet their needs for energy. As we have in-

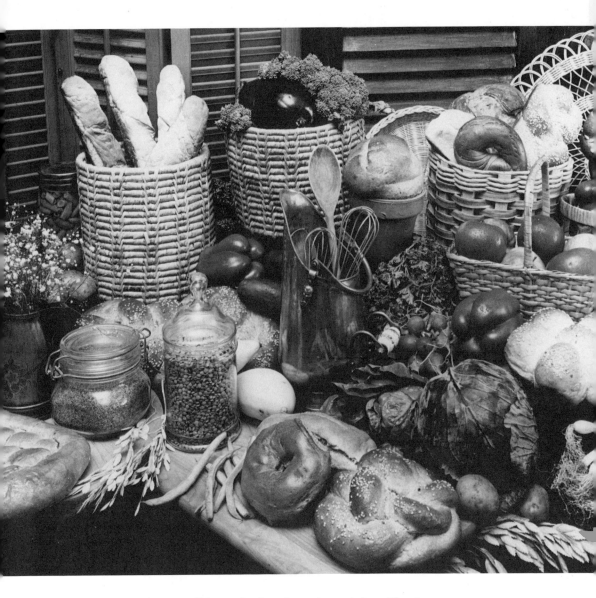

It is possible to obtain adequate protein without eating meat by combining beans and whole grains.

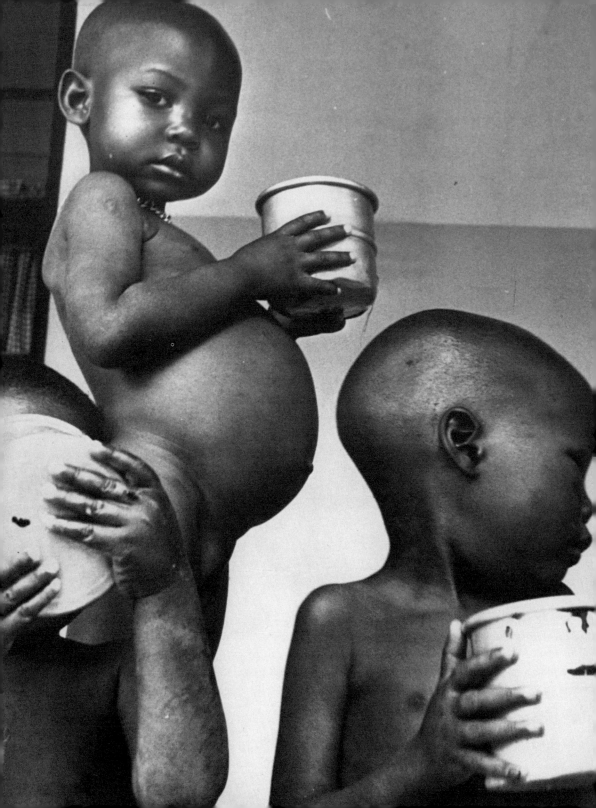

dicated, however, many plants (but not all) are poor in protein. If insufficient protein is available from either plant or animal sources, it is likely that people will suffer a protein deficiency called *kwashiorkor*. *Kwashiorkor* means "swollen belly" in Swahili, an African language. This type of malnutrition was first studied intensively in Africa. People with kwashiorkor don't look like they are starving because they have large bellies and, often, puffy faces. To many people, they look well fed. The problem these people have is due to two factors: the availability of adequate carbohydrates (sugars) and the unavailability of proteins. Because there are adequate carbohydrates, their blood sugar levels remain near normal, nonstarvation levels. This means that there is only a modest production of insulin and glucagon. Normally, when a person begins starvation, the pancreas secretes more glucagon, and the glucagon stimulates the fat cells to release fatty acids and the muscle cells to release amino acids from the breakdown of proteins. Among the amino acids released are those we mentioned above as essential. All of these amino acids are used elsewhere in the body to reassemble enzymes important for normal functioning. In kwashiorkor, the low levels of glucagon do not stimulate the release of amino acids by the muscles, and so these important enzymes cannot be made. Without some of these enzymes, the body is unable to use adequately the food it does get. In many ways this situation is more serious than simple starvation.

Although many people who are suffering from total starvation are relatively healthy and have relatively normal bodily functions, people who have a protein deficiency show many abnormalities. Commonly, their livers are very fatty, suggesting a destruction of liver function. There are also very low levels of proteins in their blood.

One serious consequence of this low protein level has nothing to do with providing energy or substance for use in building enzymes. Rather, it has to do with the maintenance of a proper water balance between different parts of the body. Normally, the concentrations of protein dis-

These children are suffering from a protein deficiency disease called kwashiorkor, *which means "swollen belly" in the African language of Swahili.*

solved in the blood and those dissolved in the tissue fluids outside the blood vessels are roughly equal. In general, substances—including water and proteins—tend to move away from areas where they are in high concentration toward areas where they are in low concentration.

Consider a solution of protein in water. (We will refer to the concentration of protein in the water, but we might just as easily refer to the concentration of water.) In any given volume, the larger the amount of protein, the less water there will be. Imagine two compartments, A and B; A has a high concentration of protein, and B has a low concentration of protein. (We can also say that there is a low concentration of water in A and a high concentration of it in B.) (See Figure 2-1.) Protein will tend to move from compartment A to compartment B and water will tend to move from B to A. But in the body, proteins do not cross cell membranes very easily. If compartments A and B are separated by cell membranes or a sheet of cells, little protein is likely to move from A to B because its movement is restricted by the barrier between the compartments. However, cell membranes are more permeable to water than to protein. In our example, water would be able to move from compartment B to compartment A.

Now, let's see what this has to do with the problem of having little protein in the blood in kwashiorkor. If there is little protein in the blood compared with the amount in the tissue fluids, then water will tend to leave the blood vessels and enter the tissue spaces. When fluid accumulates in these spaces, it produces swelling; this condition is called *edema*. When there is edema, the affected parts of the body are puffy and soft because of the fluid that has accumulated there. This is why people with kwashiorkor have swollen bellies, puffy faces, and often puffy hands and feet.

Because people who have kwashiorkor also often have infections, it was once thought that infection might be the cause of the condition. Most physicians now think, however, that people with the disease are just more likely to get infections. One complication of edema is that the swelling tends to put pressure on blood vessels, reducing the blood flow in them. If there is an injury, the reduced blood flow may reduce the ability of the body to fight an infection. Normally, our bodies combat infection by means of our immune systems. Components of the immune system are transported to an infected area by being carried in the blood. But the antibodies produced by the immune system (gammaglobulins) are

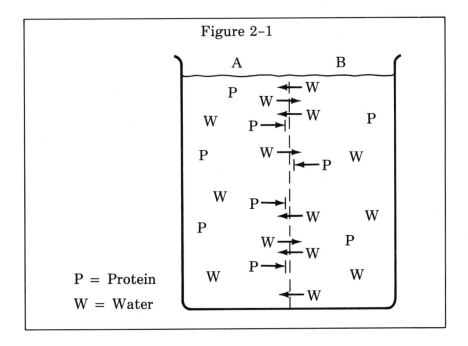

Figure 2-1

P = Protein

W = Water

proteins; since protein deficiency is widespread in this disease, there may be defects in the ability of the immune system to produce antibodies. If the blood flow is reduced, this process may not operate efficiently. In addition, if there is a lack of vitamins, especially vitamin C, wounds may not heal very well. As we shall see in chapter five, vitamin C is very important for wound healing.

Finally, when there is an infection, there also is often a fever. The fever helps the body fight the infection in several ways, but more food must be burned to provide the heat that produces the increase in body temperature. We have already stated that people with this disease have trouble making enough enzymes to support their ordinary levels of metabolic activity. As you might imagine, infections may make people with kwashiorkor, who are living on marginal diets, even more susceptible to the effects of protein deficiency. Kwashiorkor illustrates just one of the ways that good nutrition is important to good health and the ability to withstand the threats posed by infectious diseases.

Chapter Four

DIABETES

Diabetes is the Greek term for "siphon." As you may know, a siphon is a tube that can be used to drain a fluid from a container. People who have diabetes pass large amounts of urine.

Two quite different diseases are included under this one term. One of them, *diabetes insipidus*, involves the production of an abundant amount of urine as a result of a deficiency in the production of a hormone (antidiuretic hormone, or ADH) by a part of the brain known as the *pituitary gland*. The other, *diabetes mellitus*, is the result of a disorder in the pancreas. The pancreas, the small gland located near the stomach that we discussed in chapter two, secretes two hormones into the blood: insulin and glucagon. In diabetes mellitus, the pancreatic cells that normally produce insulin fail to do so. The failure may be total, or it may be that the pancreas fails to produce adequate amounts of insulin.

Insulin is important in the body because when it is present, many of the cells in the body, especially fat and muscle cells, take up sugar from the blood. The main sugar found in the blood is glucose, and insulin makes it easier for glucose to cross the membranes and enter these cells. When insulin production by the pancrease decreases, glucose accumulates in the blood. If it reaches high concentrations in the blood, it will be lost in the urine.

There are also two types of diabetes mellitus. Logically, these are named Type I and Type II. Type I is also called Insulin Dependent Diabetes Mellitus (or IDDM). This type of diabetes usually develops suddenly in younger people, often at about the time of puberty. It has been claimed that its onset is associated with viral infections, though there is no general agreement on this point. In such persons, the pancreas fails completely in its ability to produce insulin, and so Type I diabetics must take insulin regularly; otherwise severe complications of the disease develop, ending in death.

Type II is also called Non-Insulin Dependent Diabetes Mellitus (or NIDDM). As the name suggests, people with Type II disease are not totally dependent on taking extra insulin. In these people, the pancreas still produces insulin but does so in inadequate amounts. Type II diabetes usually first appears in people aged fifty or sixty, and its onset is gradual. The severity of the condition varies among different individuals. Most of these people produce some insulin, but sometimes they must receive additional amounts in order to achieve normal levels in the blood. If they do not take insulin, they develop high blood sugar levels and excrete sugar in their urine, but they do not develop the severe symptoms characteristic of Type I and are not at immediate risk of dying.

How does this condition lead to the production of large volumes of urine? The organ responsible for regulating the amount of water in the body, and for the elimination of waste materials resulting from metabolic activity, is the kidney. Normally, a little glucose is lost from the blood to the kidney tubules that produce the urine. In most people, this small amount of glucose is reabsorbed by the kidney and returned to the blood, so very little is left in the urine after it passes through the tubule and into the bladder for elimination from the body. In people with diabetes, however, so much sugar is lost to the kidney tubules that the mechanisms for reabsorbing it cannot keep up and sugar is lost in the urine. The term *mellitus* refers to honeybees; it was applied to this form of diabetes in the late 1600s after a physician named Willis noted that the urine was sweet "as if imbued with honey and sugar."

Part of the reason why a person with diabetes mellitus eliminates so much urine is that the person drinks large amounts of water. To under-

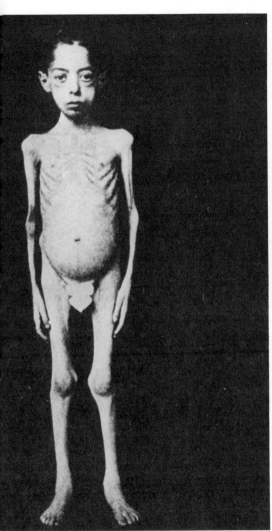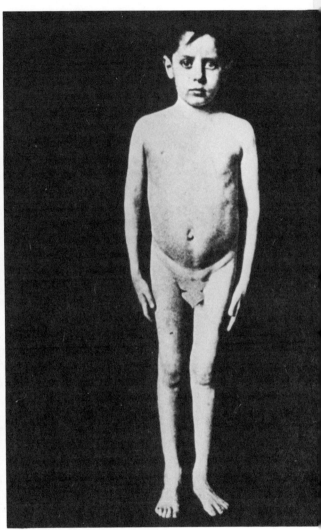

On the left is a 1922 photograph of a diabetic child
before treatment with insulin; on the right, a photo of the
same child taken two months after treatment began.

stand why, we need to return to the fact that the blood sugar level is high. When a liquid has a large amount of material dissolved in it, it is said to have a high osmotic strength. This means that if it is placed next to another body of water that contains a smaller amount of the material, and if the barrier between these two bodies permits the passage of water but not of the materials dissolved in them, then water will flow from the one that has less dissolved material to the one that has more. This process is called *osmosis*. (You might find it helpful to refer to our discussions of osmosis in chapters three and eight.) Blood always contains a little less than 1 percent salt. When it also contains more sugar than normal, it has a higher osmotic strength than normal. This means that water will tend to flow out of the body cells into the blood. The very same thing happens when a person suffers from a lack of drinking water, and for basically the same reason.

Cells in a part of the brain near the pituitary are especially sensitive to this loss of water, and these cells appear to be responsible for producing drinking behavior. In a person who simply lacks water, this results in a replacement of the missing water and correction of the problem. In a person with a high blood sugar level, it results in an increase in blood volume (an increase in the total amount of liquid inside the blood vessels), which in turn tends to produce an elevation of blood pressure. A result of all of this is that the kidney operates to restore the blood volume or pressure by excreting large amounts of urine, which eliminates fluid from the blood. This is one reason why diabetics produce a large volume of urine containing a large amount of sugar.

Since the loss of this sugar represents the loss of a source of energy, it is potentially a serious problem. Some of the sugar comes from stores within the body, and some comes from the conversion of other materials in the body to sugar. The earliest description of diabetes (in about A.D. 200 by the Greek physician Aretaeus of Cappadocia) characterized it as "a melting down of the flesh and limbs into urine." In a way this is what happens, though of course the flesh does not melt in the usual sense.

There are other problems for the person who has diabetes, too. One is that the blood tends to become more acidic. The reasons why are very complicated and are not entirely understood. When the amount of insulin produced by the pancreas is low, the amount of sugar in the blood is high, as we have already learned. Normally, a high level of sugar in the blood suppresses the pancreas, so that it does not release glucagon. In diabetic persons, however, the high levels of glucose in the blood do not suppress the release of glucagon. In the blood of diabetics, therefore, there tend to be high levels of glucagon and low levels of insulin. The low levels of insulin favor the loss of stores from fat cells.

As we noted in chapter two and shall encounter again in chapter eleven, fat cells release fatty acids, which travel in the blood to the liver. In the liver, the fatty acids are normally converted to a number of different substances. When the concentrations of both glucose and glucagon are high, however, the liver tends to produce an excess of substances called ketones. Ketones serve as an important fuel for brain and muscle, especially during starvation, but under these conditions they are produced in such large quantities that the tissues cannot keep up with the supply, and so their concentration in the blood rises. In persons with very low levels of insulin and high levels of ketones in the blood, the breath has a pleasant smell, similar to that of a chemical known as acetone, which is another ketone. The loss of ketones in the urine and from the breath also represents the loss of an energy source.

Another problem is that the fatty acids and the ketones are weak acids, and their presence causes the blood to become more acidic. When a person exercises, one of the chemicals often produced in the muscles is lactic acid, another kind of acid. The response of the body to acid conditions in the blood is to increase the breathing rate. As you might guess, this is exactly what is needed to provide more oxygen during exercise, and so the response of the body is appropriate for these conditions. The response of a person suffering from a lack of insulin and from too many acids and ketones in the blood is the same: heavy breathing. The heart also responds with an increase in its rate. If untreated, a lack of insulin can lead to shock, a loss of consciousness, coma, and death.

Yet another problem that often accompanies diabetes is a high frequency of heart disease, due to accumulations of fatty material in the coronary blood vessels, the blood vessels that supply the heart muscle itself. Physicians have identified a number of so-called risk factors associated with this type of heart disease. Among these factors are high blood pressure and high levels of fats, especially triglycerides and cholesterol, in the blood. In general, persons with diabetes tend to have these conditions.

Even when these risks are taken into account, an unknown "diabetic factor" appears to be responsible for the fact that diabetic persons have a greater chance of having severe problems than do nondiabetics with the same levels of these risk factors. Nondiabetic women have a much lower chance of developing heart disease than do men. Both diabetic men and diabetic women have a greater chance of developing heart disease than do nondiabetic members of the same sex. It is also true that women seem to suffer more severely than do men if both are diabetic and both have the same levels of these risk factors. Consequently, diabetic women are about as likely to develop these problems as are diabetic men; the relative advantage that women usually have over men disappears when there is diabetes in both.

No one knows just why this is so. It is important to point out that diabetes alone does not appear to be the cause of the increased risk. Studies of people in Japan and in Africa indicate that the incidence of heart disease is about the same for diabetics as for nondiabetics. Physicians and scientists interpret these findings to mean that diabetes does not itself cause the increased risk of heart disease. If the risk factors mentioned above are present, however, then diabetes appears to cause their effects to be more severe. This is a good sign. It suggests that diabetics can greatly decrease their risk of heart disease if their diabetes can be managed properly and if they can control the factors that nondiabetic heart patients attempt to control.

There is still another general threat to health that often accompanies diabetes, though it is more severe if the diabetes is either untreated or poorly treated: the problem of infections. This general problem is too large to attempt to cover it here, but a brief consideration of one way in which infection becomes a problem in persons with diabetes may help to make the point. When their diabetes is not well managed, for reasons that are not yet clear people often experience a deterioration in the functions of the nerves supplying the extremities, especially the feet. Two parts of the nervous system are often affected. One part is the *sensory system*, which normally provides sensations of touch, pressure, and pain in the skin. The other is the so-called *sympathetic nervous system*, which is involved in the regulation of blood flow through the small arteries. When the sensory system's monitoring of conditions in the skin of the feet is reduced, small injuries (ingrown toenails, blisters) may go unnoticed for some time. A callus, or thickening of the skin, may also develop. Ordinarily when calluses develop to such a size and hardness that they become a problem, a person is aware of their presence and so changes his or her step so that most of the load is transferred to other parts of the foot. This causes calluses to develop elsewhere but relieves the pressure and, eventually, the size of a hardened callus. If the callus really becomes a problem, the person seeks medical assistance. In the untreated diabetic with a nervous system dysfunction, these small injuries often go unrecognized. Any break in the skin may serve as a route through which bacteria or other organisms can enter the body and establish an infection. In the diabetic, because of problems with the regulation of blood flow due to the deterioration of the sympathetic nervous system, the blood circulation is often poor. This favors the development of a severe infection, because the body is unable to bring enough blood to the area to fight the invading organisms, yet the blood that does arrive is rich in sugars, which may serve as an energy source for the bacteria. Unfortunately, diabetics often fail to respond well to treatment with antibiotics, and it sometimes becomes necessary to amputate parts of the extremity.

Fortunately, the treatment of diabetes (both Types I and II) is fairly simple, although it requires care and attention to detail to prevent minor problems from becoming big ones. Insulin is now available at low cost; it is administered by injection (usually self-injection). Injected insulin performs the same role as that produced normally by the pancreas. Some care is required, however, because the injected insulin is present in high concentrations shortly after it is administered, and then its level declines gradually. Some types of natural insulin enter the blood very slowly. A person on insulin, therefore, must always take the same type of insulin (unless otherwise directed by a physician) and must be careful about the amount that is taken, the time of day at which it is taken, and his or her pattern of eating and activity throughout the day. Taking too little insulin or eating inappropriately produces the problems of untreated diabetes. Taking too much insulin can also be a serious problem: insulin causes cells to take up glucose from the blood. Also, the pancreas may not respond rapidly to the presence of this insulin, or to the change in blood glucose levels, by secreting glucagon. If there is too much insulin, blood sugar levels may fall very low. This is a problem because the brain depends almost exclusively on glucose for its energy supply. The brain uses glucose at a very high rate, and when the level in the blood falls too low, a person may become disoriented or confused or may even become unconscious and lapse into a coma and die. If recognized in time, this condition can be easily handled. All that is required is to raise the blood sugar level; a candy bar, a soft drink (one that contains sugar—not a diet drink with artificial sweeteners), or fruit juice can provide a dramatic recovery in minutes.

Chapter Five

THE VITAMIN DEFICIENCY DISEASES

Commenting on a certain discovery, Mark Twain once remarked that "recent findings have cast much doubt upon the subject, and if scientists continue their investigations, soon we shall know nothing about it." That statement might well apply to attempts to define vitamins. Most people know about vitamins; at least they recognize the word and appreciate that it is important to obtain vitamins in the diet. Any attempt to define the vitamins more rigorously, however, is a bit more difficult. In the process we learn what we do know and what we do not know concerning this important group of chemicals.

The vitamins include a group of compounds that are essential for life and health but that need to be present in food in only very low concentrations. Other groups also fit this definition, but they are not generally considered to vitamins. One of these groups is the trace metals: iron, cobalt, calcium, cadmium, zinc, and various others. Vitamins can be distinguished from these on the basis of chemical structure: vitamins are organic molecules, that is, they are complex molecules built mostly from carbon, hydrogen, oxygen, and nitrogen. As we saw in chapter two, there are other organic molecules besides vitamins that need be present in only small amounts, for example the essential amino acids. How can we distinguish the vitamins from these? In general, vitamins are needed in far smaller quantities than are the essential amino acids and they are not incorporated into the structure of the body. But to some extent, our definition of vitamins is a bit arbitrary.

The vitamins are not just found in our foods. Some of them are produced in our intestines by the bacteria that live there, in sufficient quantities to serve our needs. Others may be synthesized inside the body (the inside of the intestine is not really considered to be inside the body) by some animals but not by others. Humans synthesize vitamin D, for example, and most animals synthesize at least some vitamin C.

Table 2 lists the vitamins by name and by their letter designation. Notice that the vitamins are listed in two groups: the fat-soluble and the water-soluble vitamins. As these terms suggest, the first group dissolves in fats but not in water, and the second group dissolves in water but not in fats. The fat-soluble vitamins can be stored in the body, but the water-soluble ones cannot. Because the fat-soluble vitamins can be stored, excessive levels of some of these, especially vitamins A and D, sometimes build up. High levels of vitamin A are associated with skin and joint problems, and high levels of vitamin D result in the accumulation of calcium deposits in some of the soft organs, especially the lungs and kidneys.

All the known vitamins have now been synthesized in the laboratory, and we have a good understanding of how many of them function in the body. In general, the B vitamins serve as *coenzymes*; that is, they assist enzymes in speeding chemical reactions. Vitamin B_1 (thiamine), for example, breaks down fatty acids into two-carbon fragments that can then be combined with other chemicals and used to provide energy. This is the main route by which we obtain energy from our stored fats. Vitamin B_2 plays an important role in some of the chemical steps that come after those that depend on vitamin B_1. Vitamin B_6 is very important in protein metabolism, where it participates in a wide variety of chemical reactions that serve to transfer parts of molecules between different amino acids and to remove or to add components to amino acids and proteins.

Vitamin B_{12} is found only in a few animal sources, especially liver and kidney. It is almost entirely absent from plants. No one knows exactly where or how the vitamin found in animal tissues is produced, though we do know that it is produced by some bacteria. The minimum require-

TABLE 2
The Vitamins

Fat-Soluble			Water-Soluble	
Letter	*Name*		*Letter*	*Name*
Vitamin A	Retinol		Vitamin B_1	Thiamine
Vitamin D	Calciferol		Vitamin B_2	Riboflavin
Vitamin E	-Tocopherol		Vitamin B_3	Niacin
Vitamin K	Phylloquinone		Vitamin B_6	Pyridoxine
			Vitamin B_5	Pantothenic Acid
			Vitamin B_8 (H)	Biotin
			Vitamin B_c (M)	Folic Acid
			Vitamin B_{12}	Cobalbumin
			Vitamin C	Ascorbic Acid

ments for B_{12} are not known, nor are details of the mechanism by which the vitamin works.

A vitamin with a rather unusual type of function in the body is vitamin E. Vitamin E appears to have an important role in preventing some of the effects of oxidation in the body. Ordinarily, we think of oxygen as important to life. Since it is required for the efficient use of our foods as a source of energy, oxygen certainly is important. Some compounds in the body, however, are quite sensitive to the levels of oxygen present. For example, many fats are rapidly altered in the presence of oxygen, and vitamin A, which is important for vision, is destroyed in the presence of high levels of oxygen.

Though we have a good understanding of the chemical nature of the vitamins and know a great deal about what many of them do in the body, there is a large gap in our understanding of how the lack of any one vitamin actually causes the symptoms that are produced. This may be because we don't know which of the things a vitamin does in the body is most important, at least for preventing the appearance of the diseased

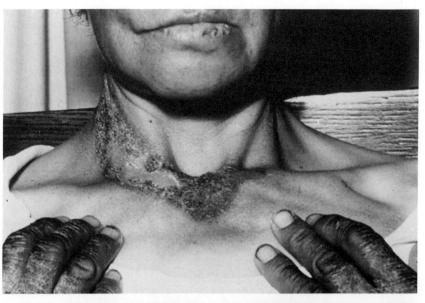

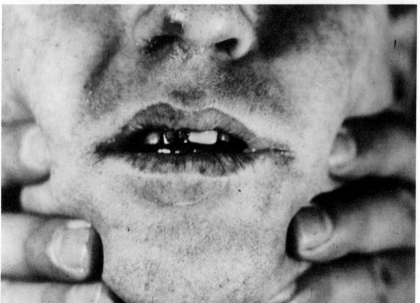

condition that results from a lack of the vitamin. It may also be due to the fact that we do not know all of the things that each vitamin does. Still, it seems remarkable that the lack of two vitamins, niacin and riboflavin, both of which act on very nearly the same biochemical processes, should cause such apparently different diseases as pellagra—due to niacin deficiency—and the wide variety of skin, eye, and mouth problems that accompany diets with insufficient riboflavin.

VITAMIN A

Let us begin our consideration of deficiency diseases with one of the vitamins for which the basis of disease is better known: vitamin A (retinol). A lack of this important vitamin causes two types of problems that are very well understood. Vitamin A is the compound from which the molecule called *rhodopsin* is made. To understand the importance of this molecule, we need to know that our eyes have two types of cells, called *receptor cells*, that respond to light. One type, the rods, responds to light of any color. The other, the cones, are responsible for color vision. There are three types: those sensitive to red, to blue, and to green. The rods contain rhodopsin, and it is the absorption of light by rhodopsin that is the first event in "seeing" with the rods. Because the rod cells are more sensitive to light than the cones are, we use the rod cells for night vision. You do not see colors outdoors at night because the cones responsible for color vision are not receiving enough light to be activated. If a person suffers a vitamin A deficiency, there will not be enough rhodopsin produced, and the rods will not function properly, causing night blindness.

A second problem that is well understood is that there is a failure of growth in young people when diets are deficient in vitamin A. When the long bones of the arms and legs grow, they increase in length because,

Top: pellagra, a niacin deficiency disease, is marked by inflamed and ulcerated skin of the hands, arms, legs, and neck. Bottom: cracks at the corners of the mouth, inflamed lips, and purple-red tongue are signs of a riboflavin deficiency.

at each end of the bone, new bone is produced. The area in which new bone is produced is called the *epiphysis*, or growth plate. One of the actions of vitamin A in young people is to maintain growth in these regions. The hormones testosterone (in males) and estrogen (in females) also keep these regions growing. Without vitamin A, however, the rate of growth at the epiphyses decreases greatly, and so full adult height may not be attained. For the past few generations children have been growing taller than their parents. The reason seems to be that our modern diets provide more nutrients and vitamins than those of older generations, so that young people today are probably growing to about the normal limits that can be reached by humans, while their parents and grandparents did not reach full adult size because of a lack of both nutrients and vitamins. The Japanese have been quite small people for several generations. Since World War II, however, children in Japan have been growing at rates that are beginning to match those of Americans and Europeans. This suggests that the same phenomenon has been occurring in Japan in recent times.

Other aspects of vitamin A deficiency are less well understood. A deficiency of vitamin A often results in scaly skin, increased susceptibility to infection, and failures of the reproductive function. All these conditions may be related: any reduction in the integrity of the *epithelia*, or linings, will likely impair reproductive function. Skin is just one kind of epithelium; other epithelia line the respiratory tract, digestive system, blood vessels, excretory system, and reproductive system. If the integrity of the lining of any part of the body is reduced, it increases the possibility that the lining will be penetrated and that an infection will occur when it comes in contact with disease organisms. In addition, the sperm that are produced by males grow from an epithelium in the testis, and the eggs produced by the female implant in the epithelial wall of the uterus after fertilization. Vitamin A seems to help maintain the health of all these epithelia.

VITAMIN C

In the days of the sailing ships one of the most common diseases aboard ship was scurvy, a result of insufficient vitamin C. On long voyages the disease might kill half the crew. Scurvy was also prevalent on land, particularly during the winter months, when some of the foods that con-

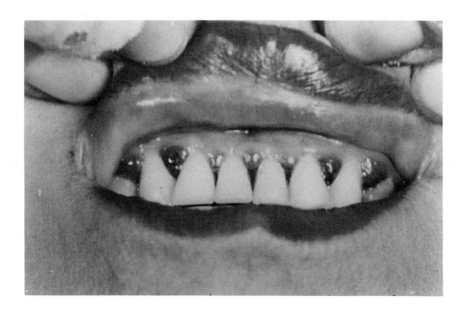

*Scurvy is characterized by swollen and
bleeding gums and loosened teeth.*

tain the vitamin were in short supply. Humans are among the few animals
that cannot synthesize this vitamin in their bodies.

A number of functions of vitamin C are known, but since they all
involve complex chemistry, we will not go into them here. But it has been
known for some time that some of the cells in the body secrete specific
types of materials that serve as a substrate, or cement, between all
individual cells. Vitamin C plays an important role in the production of
one of these materials, called *collagen*. Since many cells are anchored in,
or guided by, this substance, it is quite important for normal development.
Vitamin C is also important for the integrity of tissues and organs and
for the processes of wound repair. People with vitamin C deficiency often
bruise easily, apparently because collagen is poorly developed in the walls
of their blood vessels, making them fragile and subject to rupture. (It is
the leakage and pooling of deoxygenated blood in tissue spaces that make
the dark spot that we call a bruise.) In addition, scar formation, which

depends upon the production of large amounts of collagen, is impaired when vitamin C is not available in adequate amounts.

Several years ago, Dr. Linus Pauling, a Nobel Prize–winning chemist, suggested that the ingestion of large amounts of vitamin C gives protection against the common cold. It remains unclear whether this is really so, but as a result of his suggestion, many people started consuming several grams of this vitamin each day.

Some of these people found that they still caught colds and later stopped taking the vitamin. To their surprise, they often found that for a while they bruised much more easily after they stopped taking this vitamin. The phenomenon they observed is what is known as *rebound deficiency*. In chapter one, in our discussion of physiology, we noted that the body is capable of adapting to various conditions imposed upon it. Adaptation is the rule in physiology; the body adjusts to a new set of conditions imposed upon it and changes its function accordingly. For example, if you have been in the cold for a long time, normal room temperature feels warm. Similarly, persons who take large amounts of vitamin C (or any vitamin) adapt to that; the high level becomes the new norm. When the vitamin is suddenly taken in much lower amounts than previously, the body behaves as if there were a deficiency. In the case of vitamin C, this may appear as an increased tendency to bruise easily until the body readjusts to more normal levels.

VITAMIN D

We obtain vitamin D in two very different ways. First, it is obtained in the diet, although it is not very widespread in foods. It is found most abundantly in the livers of fish, but no one is sure why there is so much of it in fish livers. It is also found in milk and other dairy products and is rather abundant in eggs. The second way in which it is obtained is rather unusual; it is synthesized by the skin. Its synthesis requires only two conditions in normal people: sunlight on the skin and the presence of a common form of cholesterol. Under the action of sunlight in most climates, the skins of most normal adults convert enough of this form of cholesterol to vitamin D to meet all of their needs.

Vitamin D is important because of its role in helping the body to use calcium and phosphorus. It is converted into a hormone that controls the levels of at least two of the proteins that bind (combine with) calcium.

(46)

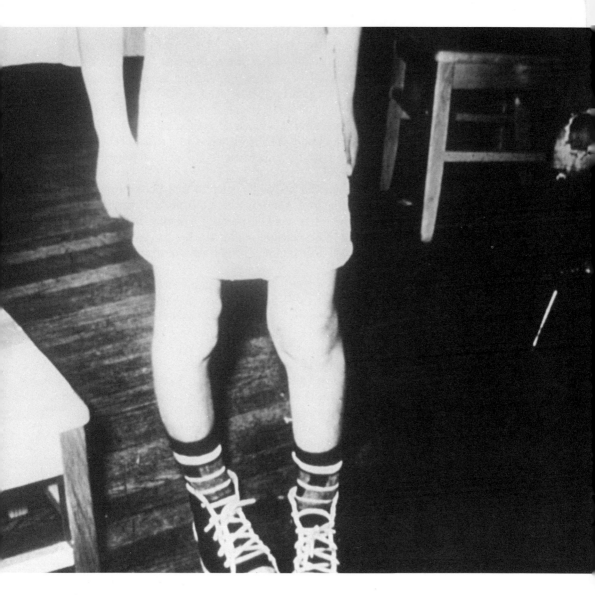

*A vitamin D deficiency produces rickets,
often characterized by bowed legs.*

Calcium, as we are coming to realize, is an extremely important substance, having many different roles. It is important for the development of the proper structure of bone, for the proper functioning of muscles and nerves, and for the control of a large number of important chemical reactions in the body. Phosphorus is now recognized as being very important in controlling the activities of the many enzymes in the body. Whether or not an enzyme affects the rate of a chemical reaction depends on whether or not there is phosphorus attached to it. Both calcium and phosphorus appear to be vitally important to the proper functioning of all of the cells in the body.

Vitamin D also helps the body use calcium and phosphorus by increasing their absorption from the intestines. Vitamin D promotes the uptake of calcium by bone as well, especially growing bone, and this process is important because calcium makes the bones strong and hard. Vitamin D also increases the removal of phosphorus from the body by the kidney.

Most of the problems experienced by humans and animals with insufficient vitamin D appear to be related more to calcium than to phosphorus. Just as the fat stored in the body serves as a reservoir of energy during times of starvation, so the skeleton serves as a reservoir for calcium during times of calcium shortage (which are comparatively rare) or during times of vitamin D shortage (which are less rare, at least in children, who often require vitamin D in their diet to support the normal growth of bones). Vitamin D deficiency produces rickets. The most obvious sign of this condition in children is the swelling of the epiphyses, the parts of bones where growth occurs. In these regions where new bone is produced, the swelling appears to be a response of the bone to a lack of available calcium. The bones of the skull, ribs, and legs (especially the knees) often show the greatest swelling, and these indicate to the physician that rickets may be responsible. Often, because the bones are softened without calcium, the legs are bowed, another characteristic sign of the disease. If a child lacks vitamin D for very long, growth is very

A scanning electron micrograph (SEM)
of a blood clot being formed by
fibrin, an elongated, ropelike protein.

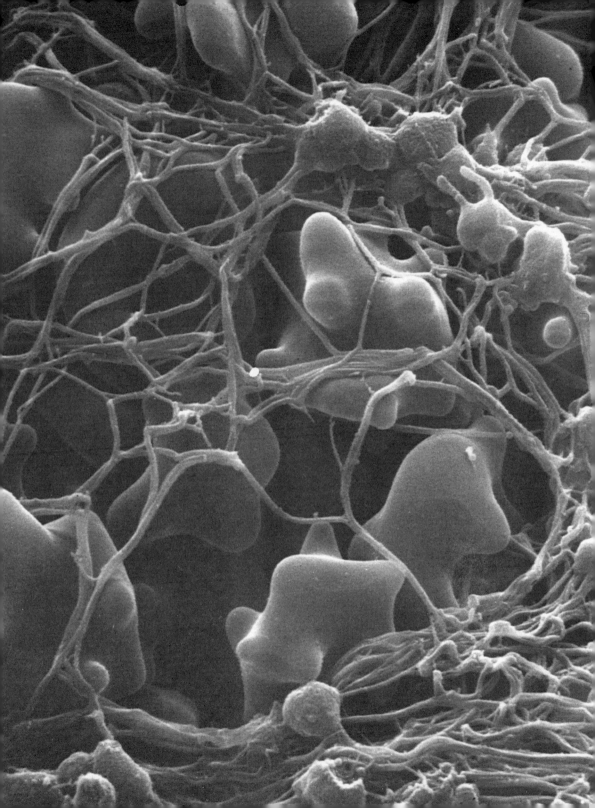

much reduced. In adults a lack of this important vitamin also weakens the bones, though, as we have seen, most adults can synthesize all they need if their skin can be exposed to reasonable amounts of sunlight.

VITAMIN K

Vitamin K is important for normal clotting of the blood. It is synthesized by bacteria that are normally present in the large intestine, and so deficiencies of this vitamin are rare. Most often, vitamin K deficiencies occur in people whose intestinal bacteria have been depleted as a result of antibiotic medications taken to combat pathogenic (disease-causing) bacterial infections.

Blood clotting involves a fairly complex series of steps, but we may understand the role of vitamin K by considering just the general mechanism of this process. First, damage to a blood vessel leads to the formation of a substance known as prothrombin activator. Prothrombin activator is an enzyme that catalyzes the conversion of a protein called *prothrombin* into another called *thrombin*. The thrombin serves as an enzyme that aids in the conversion of a protein called *fibrinogen* into *fibrin*. Fibrin is a filamentous protein that traps blood cells and begins the formation of the clot that blocks the flow of blood from the damaged blood vessel. The role of vitamin K is very simple; it is required by the liver for the synthesis of prothrombin. Without prothrombin in the blood, clotting fails to occur.

Chapter Six

ARTERIOSCLEROSIS

Before we begin this topic, it would be wise to devote some consideration to several frequently misused terms. First, the suffix *sclerosis* can stand alone as a perfectly good noun; it refers to a hardening, usually as a result of inflammation. Usually, this term is applied to hardening in either the nervous system or the circulatory system. *Arteriosclerosis* is a contraction of two words: *arterial sclerosis*. As the name suggests, this is a hardening of the arteries. *Arteriosclerosis* is a general term that includes three different kinds of conditions: *arteriolosclerosis*, *atherosclerosis*, and *Mönckeberg's arteriosclerosis*. Arteriolosclerosis is easily understood by recognizing that the name includes a contraction of *arteriole*; arterioles are the smaller arteries into which larger arteries branch. In this disease, the blood vessels that harden are the smaller arteries rather than the larger ones. Atherosclerosis affects a part of the artery called the *intima*. Arteries are made up of several layers of tissue, each wrapped around the other; the intima is the innermost layer. In atherosclerosis, it degenerates and becomes swollen and hardened, forming a structure called an *atheroma*. Often a variety of fats, including cholesterol, become deposited at these sites in both large and medium-size arteries, producing the condition called atherosclerosis. Finally, Mönckeberg's arteriosclerosis is a condition in which large quantities of calcium are deposited in the middle layers of the arteries.

In its several forms, arteriosclerosis and the complications arising from it are the leading cause of death in adults in the United States. To understand why this condition is so serious, we need to know a little about the ways in which the circulatory system works. Most of us know that the heart is the pump that moves the blood through all the blood vessels. As it leaves the heart, blood from the right side passes into the large pulmonary arteries that go to the lungs, and blood from the left side goes into the dorsal aorta and then to the rest of the body. Because the walls of these vessels are flexible, they expand when blood is forced into them, and they contract during the period when the heart is relaxed and filling with blood.

The flexibility of the large arteries does several important things. First, it reduces the back-pressure on the heart during the power stroke by giving the blood a wider vessel to pass through. Second, because the back-pressure is reduced, the load on the heart is eased so that less force is needed to deliver a given volume of blood in a given amount of time. Third, the flow of blood through the rest of the circulation is smoothed considerably, so that the flow of blood is relatively even.

What does all this have to do with the forms of arteriosclerosis? Imagine for a moment that the dorsal aorta, which carries blood to all parts of the body except the lungs, stays the same size but hardens, losing its elasticity. The advantages described above would be lost, and the output of the heart would be reduced. The body, and especially the brain, needs a constant supply of blood to remain healthy and functioning. If an adequate blood supply is not available, a wide variety of mechanisms increase the blood pressure and the output of the heart. The muscles in the walls of the arteries contract, reducing the size of the arteries and increasing the pressure. This in turn makes it harder for the heart to pump the blood into the arteries, and so it contracts more strongly. All this serves to raise the blood pressure. High blood pressure has been called "the silent killer." Perhaps the name is a bit dramatic, but it is true that persons with abnormally high blood pressure tend to suffer more heart attacks and more strokes than do people with lower blood pressures.

Why does high blood pressure increase these risks? There are at least two major parts to the answer. First, with a higher blood pressure the flow of blood in the arteries tends to be faster and more turbulent. Second, the presence of atheromas in the arteries reduces the size of the space available for blood flow and presents the possibility that some of the fatty material in the atheroma will break off and be carried along with the blood. This is more likely when the pressure is high and the flow of blood is turbulent. A solid piece of material loose in the arteries is going to get stuck somewhere, because the large arteries branch into smaller ones, and these branch into still smaller arterioles; the arterioles eventually branch into very thin, narrow vessels called *capillaries*. The capillaries are so small that even the blood cells must bend a bit in going through them. When a loose piece of atheroma finally reaches a vessel that is too small for it to go through, it plugs the vessel and interrupts the blood flow to the tissues it supplies.

This is a potentially serious matter almost anyplace in the body, but it is especially serious when the affected tissue is the brain or the heart. When the brain is affected, the result is a *stroke*. A stroke may involve a small, localized numbness or paralysis; it may cause an inability to speak or to understand speech or writing; it may cause paralysis of large portions of the body; or it may cause death, depending on the part of the brain affected and on the amount of tissue that loses its blood supply. When the heart is affected, the result is a heart attack or *coronary*. The heart is a muscle and muscle is living tissue; it must itself receive an adequate blood supply. The blood vessels that carry blood to the heart muscle itself are called the *coronary vessels*. These vessels fill with blood when the heart chambers themselves are filling with blood, but the blood in the coronary vessels comes from the dorsal aorta. If one of the coronary vessels becomes plugged, the muscle supplied by that vessel cannot continue to function and may die. If the amount of heart muscle that is affected is very large, the heart becomes less effective as a pump. If the damaged heart can no longer meet even the minimal needs of the body, death is inevitable unless appropriate medical assistance is obtained immediately.

Despite the danger of arteriosclerosis to human health, we are still far from understanding how the arteries become diseased. Part of the problem is that it is difficult to know what is cause and what is effect. For example, it is known that an atheroma involves the attachment of *platelets* to the interior of an artery. Platelets are the parts of blood cells that produce clots. Clots help to stop bleeding from wounds. But in the

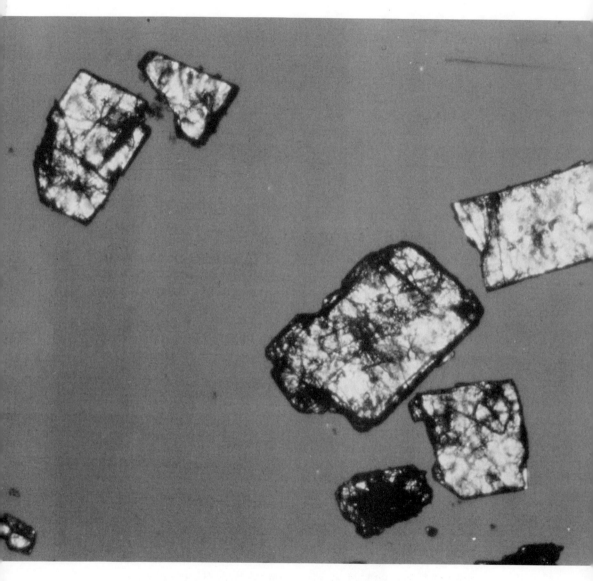

A highly magnified photo of cholesterol. Since it is a fat, it does not dissolve in water or blood.

production of atheromas, it is not known whether the platelets are responding to a pre-existing condition on the interior of the vessel or whether there is an abnormality in the activity of the platelets, so that they rupture in response to normal conditions and thus begin the process of formation of the atheroma.

A variety of factors are often associated with arterial disease. Chief among these is a high level of *cholesterol*, a type of fat, in the circulation. Cholesterol is found in many foods (for example, in egg yolks), and it is also synthesized in the body. Cholesterol is very important because it forms the backbone of many hormones (see chapter one for a description of hormones). Since cholesterol is a fat, it does not mix or dissolve in water or blood. In the blood, it is transported by being combined with proteins. Two general types of protein serve this role: low-density lipoprotein (LDL) and high-density lipoprotein (HDL). Of these two, the LDL seems to be the best indicator of the amount of cholesterol in the blood and of the risk of atherosclerosis and heart disease. For many people, the amount of cholesterol in the blood, and the risk of heart attacks, can be reduced by limiting the amount of cholesterol in the diet.

Females have less LDL in their blood than do males of the same age; and they suffer fewer problems with arterial and heart diseases. Arteriosclerosis is increasingly common with advancing age. There is some evidence that a person's susceptibility is inherited, at least in part. It is not clear why atheromas form in some places within the arteries and not in others; nor is it clear where the fats found in these plaques originate.

Arterial diseases also affect people from different cultures and of different races in different ways. People in the British Isles tend to have a high incidence of arterial disease, while people in Japan tend to have a much lower incidence. In the United States, black people tend to have a higher incidence of the disease—and of high blood pressure—than do white people. It is not clear whether these findings reflect differences in diet, life-style, racial origin, or other factors yet to be identified.

Happily, there are several aspects of the disease that are known and that can be controlled. A change in diet can reduce the levels of fats in the circulation and reduce the chances of having a heart attack or stroke. Exercise pursued wisely—and under a physician's care if there has been a prolonged period of relative inactivity—can also alter the circulating levels of fats. Exercise can also strengthen the heart and blood vessels, and it strengthens the rest of the muscles in the body, as well. These play an important role in returning blood to the heart. When exercise stops, or when a person returns to the old diet (from one designed to reduce fats), a return to high levels of fats in the circulation can be observed in as little as two weeks.

In recent years the incidence of arterial disease has decreased, possibly reflecting a greater awareness of the importance of the problem and the roles of diet and exercise by the general population. Let us hope this trend continues.

Chapter Seven

PHENYLKETONURIA

When we think of nutritional diseases, we often think of diseases that result from a lack of some required substance in the diet. For example, in the chapter on vitamin-deficiency diseases we saw that a lack of several vitamins produced characteristic problems. Most of these problems arise because the body needs that vitamin in order to perform one or more chemical reactions. Chemical reactions in the body depend on enzymes; if an enzyme or coenzyme is not present, the ability of the body to produce certain chemicals, or to use certain nutrients, may be impaired. However, problems can also occur because of the accumulation of a substance that is usually converted to another by the missing enzyme. There are many nutritional diseases that are a result of this kind of inborn error of metabolism, but we shall consider just one: phenylketonuria (PKU).

Phenylketonuria is an inherited disease caused by the lack of a specific liver enzyme. The enzyme that is missing, or present in low concentrations, is called *phenylalanine hydroxylase*. Normally, it converts one amino acid (phenylalanine) into another (tyrosine). The disease takes its name, and is diagnosed, from the abnormally high levels of phenylalanine and related compounds that are excreted in the urine. The high levels in urine come from high blood levels of these compounds. In PKU, major complications result from the accumulation of phenylalanine and related compounds rather than from a lack of tyrosine, which can be obtained in the diet. Treatment of this condition is, therefore, relatively simple: it involves the prevention of the accumulation of phenylalanine by restricting the amounts of it in the diet. This certainly requires some care, but it is an effective way to minimize the seriously harmful effects of the untreated condition. Untreated, phenylketonuria leads to convulsions and severe mental retardation.

Early recognition of PKU is necessary, however, and treatment must begin within the first two months of life if development is to be normal; otherwise an irreversible retardation appears. Although the incidence of this disease is fairly low (approximately one in every 10,000 to 20,000 births), its severity and the ease with which it can be detected and corrected have led all developed countries to test for it routinely at birth.

The diet may be returned to normal or near normal later in life, possibly as early as at age five, though there is some disagreement about this figure; some argue that the restricted diet should be continued until at least age ten. The diet can be changed probably because brain maturation is largely completed before adolescence, so the brain is less susceptible to the damaging effects of these compounds.

Chapter Eight

WATER AND SALT BALANCE

Sometimes we overlook the common things that are most important to us and fail to appreciate their importance. Water is one such item. The importance of water to living things cannot be overemphasized. All active, living things depend upon it.

Most of us know that the chemical designation for water is H_2O (or H-O-H), meaning that it has two hydrogen atoms and one oxygen atom. Water molecules are loosely linked to each other, both as liquid water and as ice. The same forces that link water molecules together make it possible for salts, such as sodium chloride ($NaCl$) or common table salt, to dissolve in it. The $NaCl$ separates into two particles called *ions*, having opposite electrical charges (Na^+ and Cl^-). Because of their interaction with water molecules, these particles are free to move at random within a body of water—this is largely why salt water conducts electricity so well. Water, therefore, acts as a good solvent for salts such as sodium chloride.

Similarly, it also acts as a good solvent for other salts and for many of the materials our body uses as nutrients and produces as waste products. The water molecule can also break into separate parts, so that H-O-H becomes H^+ and OH^-. Notice the opposite electrical charges (+

and −) on the hydrogen (H^+) and hydroxyl (OH^-) ions. The concentration of the hydrogen ions is a measure of the acidity of the water. Acidic waters have a higher concentration of hydrogen (H^+) ions. Water also has a high heat capacity, and blood—which is mostly water—effectively carries heat from the central parts of the body to the hands and feet. The evaporation of water also carries away large amounts of heat, which is helpful in cooling our bodies when we perspire.

From this brief consideration of the properties of water it is easier to understand its importance in the body. The majority of the chemical reactions that keep us alive occur in the water found throughout our bodies. Water also serves as the vehicle for transporting nutrients and wastes in the blood and from the blood to the cells.

The amount of water in the body tends to be very carefully regulated. When there is too little, a thirst center in the brain promotes drinking, so that water is replaced. The only other source for water in the body is our metabolism. Two of the products that appear when we break down our food are carbon dioxide and water. For every hundred Calories of heat produced, twelve milliliters of water are produced, on average. Although this is enough to meet the needs of some desert animals, humans need additional water from drinking.

Water is lost through the kidneys, skin, and lungs. The kidneys control the amount of water lost in the urine, and also control the concentration of the various salts in the blood. A hormone called *antidiuretic hormone*, or ADH for short, is produced by the pituitary, a small gland at the base of the brain. This hormone acts on a part of the kidney tubule, called the *collecting tubule*, that is very important in concentrating the urine. By means of other activities in the kidney, a large concentration of salt (mainly sodium chloride) is produced. As it carries urine out of the kidney, the collecting duct passes right through this region of high salt concentration. The walls of the collecting tubule are not permeable to salt, so very little flows into the tubule. But the walls are permeable to water. This means that water flows out of the tubule. Since this process leaves less water in the tubule, its salt and urea contents are concentrated. In this way, the kidney permits the body to rid itself of wastes (urea and a few other substances) in a fairly small amount of water.

Antidiuretic hormone acts to increase the permeability of the collecting tubule to water. The hormone is released by the pituitary when the amount of water in the body decreases. By increasing the ability of water to leave the collecting duct and be reabsorbed by the blood, there will be less lost in the urine, thus saving water.

There are several abnormal conditions that generally result in losses of water. Any disease that leads to vomiting or to diarrhea results in a loss of water. The water lost in this way, however, never really entered the body, since the contents of the stomach and intestines were not absorbed into the body proper. In some forms of diarrhea, fluids may be secreted by the intestine, causing a direct loss of body water. This is part of the reason why people are advised to take plenty of fluids when they get diseases with any of these symptoms.

One of the most widespread serious diseases in the world is cholera. People with this disease have terrible diarrhea and often die. It can be treated successfully in the majority of otherwise healthy individuals just by treating the symptoms—in this case by replacing the water, minerals, and nutrients that have been lost. Since the amount of water lost can approach 30 percent of the body weight each day, stricken people must drink very large quantities of water.

Frequent urination is characteristic of diabetes. Normally, much sugar is lost to the kidney tubule when the blood passes through the kidney; it is then reabsorbed into the blood. In diabetes mellitus, the concentration of sugar in the blood is very high. As a result, so much sugar passes into the kidney tubule that it cannot all be reabsorbed. This sugar also causes large amounts of water to remain in the kidney tubule, and so the water is also lost in the urine.

The condition known as *edema* involves the abnormal distribution of water rather than its loss. Ordinarily we consider that water in the body is found in three compartments: in the blood, in the interior of cells, and in the interstitial spaces, which are outside the cells and outside the circulatory system. All the water that moves between the cells and the blood moves through the interstitial spaces. Normally, the volume of water there is quite small. In edema, however, relatively large quantities of water are found in the interstitial spaces, giving the tissues a puffy appearance and a very soft feeling, usually in the hands and feet. (In chapter three we discussed edema in people with protein-deficient diets.)

Just as important to the body as water are the salts that are dissolved in it. As we saw earlier in this chapter, salts in water dissolve to give two particles (ions) having opposite electrical charges, one positive (+) and the other negative (−). The members of such a pair are termed *co-*

ions. Many of the normal constituents of cells have such electrical charges. Proteins commonly have more negative charges than positive ones. There is a co-ion associated with each of the charges on a protein, and usually these are inorganic, meaning that they are not compounds made of carbon, hydrogen, and oxygen. The most common are potassium (K^+), sodium (Na^+), and chloride (Cl^-).

Let us take a brief look at the major ions in the body and consider a few of the problems that result from various ionic imbalances.

POTASSIUM (K^+)

Potassium is the most abundant ion inside cells. The daily requirement for this ion is higher than that for sodium, largely because the kidney, where most losses occur, is not very efficient in conserving potassium, though it is efficient in getting rid of excesses of this ion. Potassium is very abundant in virtually all foods, and so healthy individuals under normal conditions never have any problem in meeting their daily needs.

There is more potassium inside cells than there is outside. These differences in potassium concentration cause an electrical charge to develop across the cell membrane. It is as if there were a very small battery across the very thin membranes that surround each of our cells. The amount of voltage across the membrane depends on the concentrations of ions on each side of the membrane. If there is a big difference—for example, many potassium ions inside the cell and few outside—there will be a large voltage across the membrane.

As we have seen, people with diabetes produce large amounts of urine because their kidneys cannot reabsorb all the water that is lost along with the glucose. This water also contains potassium. Potassium lost in this way decreases the amount of potassium on the outside of cells, and so the voltage across the cell membrane becomes high. This is important because one of the complaints of people with diabetes is that they feel weak. Before a muscle can contract, it must normally receive a signal from a nerve. This signal causes the electrical voltage across the cell membranes of individual muscle cells to decrease. If it decreases enough, it reaches a value called *threshold*, and a series of events begins that causes the muscle to contract. If it does not reach threshold, no contraction occurs. If the voltage across the membrane is high, it is harder to reach threshold, and so a contraction is less likely. This is one of the reasons why people with diabetes sometimes feel weak. From this example, we can see how important it is for the body to be able to regulate the concentrations of these ions.

SODIUM (Na$^+$)

Sodium is the most abundant positively charged ion located outside our cells. One of its major roles in the body is in determining body fluid concentration and volume. Because the sodium ion is carefully conserved by the body, very little is lost, and so the requirement for it is quite small. Because sodium is very abundant in the earth and in living things, it is obtained in varying quantities from virtually all foods. More often than not, the body must deal with an excess of sodium rather than with an insufficient supply. Most of the sodium is lost from the body via the urine, although small amounts are also lost from perspiration, tears, and the stool.

The route of sodium through the kidney during the production of urine is complex. Under normal conditions, a large quantity of sodium passes from the blood into the kidney tubule, and then most of it is reabsorbed into the blood. The small amount of sodium that is not reabsorbed is lost with the urine. The amount of sodium lost is under the control of a hormone called *aldosterone*, which is produced by a pair of small glands near the kidney, the adrenal glands. Aldosterone causes more sodium to be reabsorbed from the kidney to the blood, so that less is lost in the urine. When there is too much sodium, the adrenal glands stop releasing this hormone and more sodium is lost. Sodium may be depleted by heavy perspiration or by persistent diarrhea and vomiting. It may also be lost by persons who produce small amounts of aldosterone as a result of defects in the adrenal glands. Usually, the loss of large amounts of sodium means that chloride and water are lost as well. When there is too much sodium—for example, from eating salty foods—water tends to be retained in the body. Some people tend to retain too much sodium, even when there is not an excess of it in the diet. This may be one of the factors responsible for hypertension (high blood pressure).

CHLORIDE (Cl$^-$)

Chloride is the main negatively charged ion found in the extracellular spaces. As for sodium, the daily requirement is rather low, again owing to efficient means of conservation in the kidney. Since chloride is the major extracellular negatively charged ion, it is abundant in virtually all foods. In general, conditions that are important in affecting the chloride concentration are also important in affecting sodium. It must be noted that in the blood there is another anion, the bicarbonate ion (HCO_3^-) that can serve as a co-ion for sodium. The bicarbonate ion is important because it results from the production of CO_2 (carbon dioxide) during metabolism and because it plays an important role in regulating the acidity of the blood. In general, the chloride ion is retained by the kidney, and bicarbonate is retained (to be lost through the lung as carbon dioxide) or excreted as a part of the mechanism the body uses to regulate the acidity of the blood. Chloride transport across the kidney tubules is affected by aldosterone and ADH, the same hormones that affect potassium and sodium transport.

Although water and salts are not nutrients in the usual sense, we can see from these examples that it is important that they be present in the diet and that they be carefully regulated in the body.

Chapter Nine

OSTEOPOROSIS: THE REDUCTION OF BONE MASS

In the mid-1980s, many persons in the United States and other developed countries have benefited from the comparatively high standard of living. Many reach their sixtieth, seventieth, eightieth, or even their ninetieth years in rather good health. But a common misfortune that befalls many older citizens is a broken bone, often the hip. In preparing to set the bone, a physician takes X-rays and often finds that, in addition to the break, the bone lacks the density of the bones of younger people and that it is quite weak. The physician often learns that the bone broke because of a minor fall or even during the course of a perfectly normal activity like getting up from a chair. We do not know all of the reasons for age-related loss of bone tissue, but there are several factors that we can identify.

Some loss of bone is normal and, apparently, unavoidable, after middle age in both men and women. For women, bone loss usually begins after menopause, the time in a woman's life when she stops menstruating. This usually occurs at about age fifty, though it can occur much earlier and may not occur until as late as fifty-five or so. The high rate of bone loss for women of this age must be considered normal, because it is shown by so many and because it is not associated with any unusual problems.

For men, bone loss usually begins a bit later in life. As for women, there is a rate at which bone is lost that must be considered normal. The normal rate of bone loss for men, however, is only about half the rate of loss for women. It is not entirely clear why either sex loses bone, and it is not known precisely why the rate of loss is higher for women than for men.

There are several factors that appear to play some role in the loss of bone by both men and women. One of the most obvious is that most people decrease the amount of physical activity as they get older. Bone responds to the forces put upon it. If those forces decrease through inactivity, the bone will respond to this change. It has also been suggested that many older people suffer from a reduction in their calcium intake. This might result from a change in diet, but even if the diet remains the same, there may be a reduction in the amount of calcium absorbed from the intestines. Supplements of vitamin D may aid in increasing the absorption of calcium from the intestine and thus raising the levels of calcium in the blood. In women who have passed menopause the production of female hormones known as *estrogens* decreases. One consequence of decreased estrogen production relates to the maintenance of bone. Small glands, known as the *parathyroid glands* because they are located near the much larger thyroid gland, produce a substance known as *parathyroid hormone*. The major action of this hormone is to remove calcium from the bones. As we saw in chapter five, calcium is a very important element in regulating the actions of many enzymes in the body. Although the action of parathyroid hormone may seem strange, it is less strange when we understand the general importance of calcium and the fact that the skeleton serves as a short-term reservoir for this element. In any case, the estrogens tend to balance the action of parathyroid hormone, reducing its effectiveness in removing calcium from bone. When estrogen levels fall, this balance is disturbed.

The value of replacing the estrogens in older women is controversial. In some women, estrogen replacement appears to reduce the rate of calium loss from the bones, but estrogens are also associated with an increase of some cancers, so this strategy must be used with some care. For both men and women, the best that can be done is to reduce the rate of bone loss, since the loss of bone appears to be irreversible once it has occurred.

Osteoporosis is simply the reduction of bone mass. There is no change in the composition of the bone; there is simply less of it. In a related

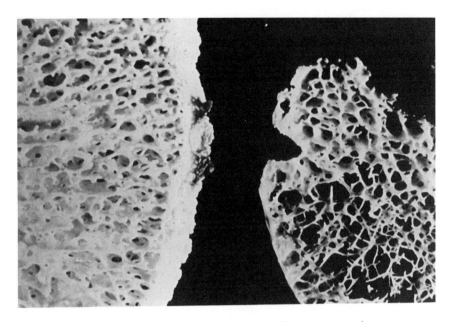

*The bone on the left is normal. The osteoporotic
bone, right, is porous, fragile, and easily broken.*

condition, *osteomalacia*, the structure of the bone stays the same but the proportion of minerals in it, mostly calcium, is reduced. Though we shall make frequent references to loss of calcium from bone during the remainder of this chapter, this refers to a reduction in the amount of whole bone, and so we are considering osteoporosis rather than osteomalacia.

As we have seen, certain rates of bone loss appear to be normal in men and women past a certain age. In some men and women, however, the rates of loss are higher than normal. Such persons are said to suffer from accelerated osteoporosis. Most of them appear to show a reduction in the absorption of calcium, though the causes of this condition are not yet clear. It may be a result of reduced production or intake of vitamin D, but it may also be due to a failure of the intestine to absorb calcium.

We have already seen that estrogen is important in females, and it is true that bone resorption and blood levels of calcium tend to be higher in women with low estrogen levels. But women with accelerated osteoporosis do not necessarily have lower levels of estrogen in their blood than women with less marked bone loss. For men the situation is even less clear. Men with osteoporosis tend to have normal hormone levels, although men with underdeveloped testes and who produce small amounts of the male hormone testosterone often have serious osteoporosis. This may be because as youths they had reduced bone formation in the first place.

Other factors associated with accelerated osteoporosis include a high intake of alcohol (which may also be associated with malnutrition), gastrointestinal surgery (with its obvious disruptive effects on intestinal function), and diabetes (although there is not an unusually high incidence of diabetes among persons with osteoporotic fractures). There are also a number of specific maladies that result in the loss of bone integrity, but we will not consider these since each represents a specific health problem with its own unique characteristics and since these affect comparatively few people.

Sometimes factors important to good health interact in ways that seem quite strange. Let us consider one such interaction. Earlier, we saw that protein deficiency might be more threatening to life than simple starvation. Curiously, diets high in protein may accelerate bone loss. Normally, excess protein is simply used for the production of energy. The protein is broken down metabolically to generate energy in much the same way that carbohydrates and fats are. As we saw, however, the nitrogen in proteins must be eliminated through the urine. This suggests that a high intake of protein will result in an increased blood flow through the kidney. If the proportion of calcium that is lost from the blood passing through the kidney remains constant, more calcium will be lost, simply because of the increased blood flow through this organ.

In addition, proteins are composed of amino acids that contain sulfur. Sulfur is lost from the body through the kidney in the form of sulfate. Normally, some of the calcium that passes from the blood into the kidney tubules is reabsorbed into the blood. The presence of sulfate reduces the amount of calcium that is reabsorbed; this is a second way in which dietary protein contributes to an increase in the loss of calcium and therefore of bone.

Phosphorus, which is also present in dietary sources of proteins, tends to reduce this effect of sulfate in the kidney, but unfortunately the presence of phosphate in the intestines also tends to interfere with the absorption of calcium from the intestines. The overall result is that a diet that is high in protein promotes a loss of calcium. In his excellent book on osteoporosis, Dr. Louis Avioli suggests that the requirement for calcium depends upon the amount of protein in the diet. He points out that the low rate of fractures in persons in developing countries, despite low calcium intake, reflects a low calcium requirement in the presence of a low intake of protein. Life never seems to be simple. When we improve living conditions so that people have a chance to grow old in good health, we find new problems that appear to be related to basic features of the aging process and of our modern life-style.

Chapter Ten

EATING DISORDERS: ANOREXIA AND BULIMIA

If physicians had only to deal with people who were identical and with conditions that could all be detected by well-defined tests, their task would be enormously simplified. Unfortunately, people are not identical, and the current state of medicine and science does not permit us to test all conditions; we don't even know the identity of all of the conditions that we might wish to test.

Among the most difficult problems are those that involve disorders of human behavior. Of such disorders we might be inclined to suggest, "Oh, it's all in the person's mind!" But the mind is a product of the functioning of the brain, and the brain is a part of the body, subject to disease and disorders like any other organ. Part of the difficulty in dealing with such disorders is that they may be very subtle—so subtle that even the person afflicted is unaware that anything is wrong.

Anorexia nervosa and *bulimia* are called eating disorders in the title of this chapter, but those who argue that they are primarily behavior disorders are probably right. The behavioral disturbance leads to disorders of nutrition. Most *anorectics* (people with anorexia) achieve their thinness by self-imposed starvation. Bulimia is generally considered to be a type of anorexia, because some anorectics are also *bulimics* (people with bulimia). Bulimia is characterized by binges of eating followed by self induced vomiting. Because vomiting is induced soon after eating, little nutritional value is obtained from the food that is eaten.

In the recent past physicians diagnosed an anorexic condition negatively, that is, on the basis of a failure to find other specific medical causes of the weight loss. Currently, several specific criteria, set forth in *The Diagnostic and Statistical Manual of Mental Disorders* (vol. 3) are used. These criteria are listed below.

Diagnostic Criteria for Anorexia Nervosa

A. Intense fear of becoming obese, which does not diminish as weight loss progresses.
B. Disturbance of body image, e.g., claiming to "feel fat" even when emaciated.
C. Weight loss of at least 25 percent of original body weight or, if under eighteen years of age, weight loss from original body weight plus projected weight gain expected from growth charts may be combined to make the 25 percent.
D. Refusal to maintain body weight over a minimal normal weight for age and height.
E. No known physical illness that would account for the weight loss.

The incidence of anorexia and bulimia appears to be increasing. In part, this is due to an increased awareness of the condition on the part of physicians, but there also appears to be a genuine increase in the number of persons affected. Some of the increase in the incidence of the disorder appears to be due to changes in social ideals. When food was less widely available than it is now in most of the developed parts of the world, stoutness was taken to be a sign of wealth and status. Eating (or behavioral) disorders of this type were largely unknown. Now, when slimness is a sign of wealth and elegance and food is so abundant as to be taken for granted, these disorders appear to be increasingly common.

Both anorexia and bulimia appear to be much more common in women than in men; from 90 to 95 percent of all patients are females. Most often, anorexia begins in adolescence, usually between the ages of twelve and twenty-five, though it may span a range of age from seven to fifty-nine. Opinions differ on whether there is a trend toward onset at younger ages;

some argue that there is an increase in all age groups. It tends to be more common in the upper socioeconomic groups. Overall, about 1 percent of all middle-class adolescent women are affected. There do appear to be patterns within families. Anorexia appears to be more likely in families where there is known depression or instances of eating disorders. Among identical twins, it is quite likely that if one twin has the condition, the other will also. Very recently (*Science*, 1986) it was reported that there appears to be a link between depression, anorexia, and a condition known as *Cushing's disease*, a pituitary-adrenal disorder. People with these diseases all have one characteristic in common: they all tend to produce excess amounts of the hormone *cortisol*.

Cortisol is often characterized as a stress hormone. It is found in persons who are under various kinds of stress. Anorexia is more common following stressful changes in schooling or in family location. When anorectics gain weight, their cortisol levels return to normal. For anorectics, it may be that the weight loss comes first and that the change in cortisol levels follows. The high cortisol levels, however, may be associated with depression and the continuance of the anorexic condition. In any case, this recent finding may eventually show the way to diagnose and treat persons with any or all of these disorders.

It is worth noting that anorexia is not always associated with negative aspects of a person's personality. For example, many anorectics achieve good grades in school. The condition is also more common in people whose profession favors slimness, such as ballet students, models, and jockeys.

Adolescence is the time when young women normally begin menstruation. If body weight decreases and body fat falls to less than 17 percent of body weight, menstruation may be abnormal, and when body fat falls to 9 percent of the body weight or less, it may stop altogether. This is, perhaps, one indication that our current preoccupation with slimness may not be consistent with what is best for our bodies. Another indication comes from the new Metropolitan Insurance Company's height/weight tables, which were prepared in 1983. These tables specify the weights of people at various heights for people who are long-lived. The values given in the 1983 tables are generally higher than those found in similar tables prepared in 1959. The new tables were criticized, partly on scientific and statistical grounds, and perhaps also because information that does not agree with our present concept that "thin is best" is immediately rejected.

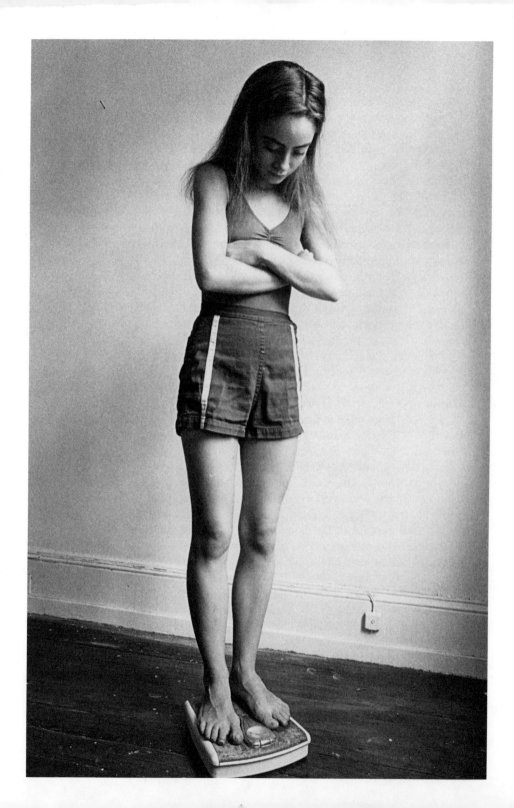

In addition to abnormalities in menstruation, people suffering from anorexia show many of the same symptoms that are shown by starving people. Obviously, one symptom is a low body weight for a given height. Another is a lowering of the vital signs, indicators that reflect the general state of health of an individual. These include a lowering of the pulse rate, blood pressure, breathing rate, and body temperature. Often there is a loss of muscle mass, as well as a loss of body fat. The levels of hormones, especially glucagon and insulin, are also altered (see chapter two), and the person tends to be inactive and slow in his or her behavior.

By itself, bulimia is a disease characterized by insatiable hunger. People may overeat for a variety of reasons. Some appear to eat simply for the pleasure of it, while others eat as a response to stress. Still others may overeat as an after-effect of diet medications. Bulimia followed by self-induced vomiting may be present in people of normal weight who are afraid of becoming fat; it may also be found in persons whose weight/height ratio approaches that of anorectics and who maintain low weight by purging all food after an eating binge. Diagnostic criteria for bulimia are given in the table below:

 Diagnostic Criteria for Bulimia

A. Recurrent episodes of binge-eating (rapid consumption of a large amount of food in a discrete period of time, usually less than two hours).
B. At least three of the following:

1. Consumption of high-caloric, easily ingested food during a binge;
2. Inconspicuous eating during a binge;
3. Termination of such eating episodes by abdominal pain, sleep, social interruption, or self-induced vomiting;
4. Repeated attempts to lose weight by severely restrictive diets, self-induced vomiting, or use of cathartics or diuretics;

Anorexia usually begins during the teen years and is marked by an intense fear of becoming fat.

5. Frequent weight fluctuations greater than ten pounds (4.5 kg) due to alternating binges and fasts.

C. Awareness that the eating pattern is abnormal and fear of not being able to stop eating voluntarily.

D. Depressed mood and self-deprecating thoughts following eating binges.

E. The bulimic episodes are not due to anorexia nervosa or any known physical disorder.

At present, excellent medical programs exist for the treatment of persons suffering from each of these eating (behavioral) disorders. Since the fatality rate for persons with these disorders averages 20 percent above that for the general population, it is important that such people get qualified help. Specific courses of action will not be outlined here because, as we have seen, there are many different aspects of each condition, and these should be diagnosed for each individual by competent medical personnel. Also, people should not be tempted into self-diagnosis and self-treatment, since it may be that there is a specific medical cause that is responsible for the symptoms.

Treatment often involves the specification of a good diet plan, with careful provision made for keeping accurate records. Sometimes psychotherapy is specified, either for the patient alone, for a group, or for the family. Ultimately, of course, the goal is to transfer responsibility back to the patient so that she or he may enjoy a long, happy, and productive life.

Chapter Eleven

OBESITY

Although the notion of *diet*, in the sense of controlling what we eat, is around us all the time in advertising and in conversation, most of us give little thought to the amount of food we eat. For most people adult body weight stays constant over a period of from thirty to forty years. Although there may be a gradual increase in weight over this period, it rarely exceeds 10 percent of body weight. If we do all the proper arithmetic and average this weight gain over the thirty-to-forty-year period, we can calculate that most people consume within about six calories the amount of energy they burn each day. Although we know a great deal about how food and the energy it contains are transferred from the intestines to various locations in the body, the basis of this excellent regulation is poorly understood.

It is well known that sensations of hunger and satiety (absence of hunger) arise from two separate centers in the brain. Both are located in the *hypothalamus*, which lies below the cerebral hemispheres and above the nasal cavity. The feeding center is located toward the sides of the hypothalamus (lateral hypothalamus). If it is damaged or destroyed, the animal or person will not eat and may starve to death. If this center is stimulated electrically by means of electrodes placed in this part of the brain, the subject eats excessively large amounts of food. The satiety center is located near the bottom of the hypothalamus along the midline (ventro-medial hypothalamus). If it is damaged or destroyed, the victim overeats. If, on the other hand, it is stimulated electrically for long periods of time, the subject will starve. Activity in each of these centers can be changed by the action of appropriate hormones. The two centers appear to communicate with each other so that only one dominates at a time.

Let us consider some of the factors that appear to affect eating, presumably through these centers in the brain. The simple sugar glucose is the only sugar present in any quantity in the blood. The brain depends on glucose almost exclusively for its considerable demands for energy. When the blood sugar level falls, as it does some hours after a meal, movements in the stomach and intestine increase. These movements often appear to lead to the sensation of hunger. Even without such movements, however, there can be strong sensations of hunger when the blood sugar levels are low. Before you conclude that blood glucose levels are the key to hunger, you should know that persons with diabetes mellitus have unusually high blood glucose levels, yet they are often hungry.

What leads to the sensation of satiety? Eating usually produces increased movement in the stomach and intestines, although both may be distended because of the food contained within them. Eating also produces a slight rise in body temperature because of the energy required to break down the food, take it up from the intestine, and convert it into various useful forms. An increase in the temperature of the hypothalamus usually produces a reduction in eating. For people who are in good health and who are reasonably well-nourished, satiety is reached after an adequate meal has been eaten. For most people, this happens about twenty minutes after eating begins, long before the meal has been digested. In short, the basis of the regulation of eating and therefore of the control of body weight is poorly understood, at least in terms of the detailed mechanisms at work.

As discussed in chapter four, the amount of glucose in the blood is under the continuous control of two hormones, insulin and glucagon, both produced and secreted by the pancreas, a small gland near the stomach. When blood glucose levels are high, the pancrease releases insulin. Insulin has little effect on the permeability of the liver and brain, but it has powerful effects on muscle and fat cells: it makes them permeable to glucose. Fat cells convert glucose into various kinds of fats, which are then stored in the cells; muscle cells convert glucose to glycogen, a form of starch. As glucose enters these cells, its concentration in the blood decreases. When blood glucose levels are low, the pancreas secretes glucagon. Glucagon stimulates the liver to convert glycogen to glucose and to release it to the blood. It also stimulates fat cells to break down some of their stored fat and to release fats into the blood. The blood carries these fats to all parts of the body, including the liver. In the liver the fats may be converted to glucose and released into the blood. Through both of these general mechanisms, glucagon serves to restore the levels of glucose in the blood.

In addition to glucagon and insulin, growth hormone, produced by the pituitary, and the sex hormones, produced by the gonads, tend to affect the levels of blood glucose. All these hormones tend to drive glucose into the various cells of the body. Since these hormones are involved in growth and maturation, it is easy to understand why they have such actions. Another hormone, epinephrine (or adrenaline), is produced in times of acute stress, that is, when the person or animal is suddenly placed in a life-threatening situation. Epinephrine acts like insulin, driving glucose into muscle cells to provide energy for the activity that usually accompanies such emergencies. Often this leaves a person quite shaky afterward. The shakiness has the same basis as the shakiness that sometimes occurs with hunger—a low blood sugar level. It has been suggested that the sensitivity of muscle cell membranes to the action of insulin in promoting the uptake of glucose may be dependent on the state of the conditioning of the muscle. That is, muscles that are exercised regularly may take up more glucose than muscles that are not exercised when both are presented with the same concentrations of glucose and insulin. If true, this could mean that weight is more easily controlled if a person is engaged in some form of exercise that conditions the muscles.

For both sexes, three different body types are recognized: ectomorphs (slender), mesomorphs (muscular), and endomorphs (obese). Individuals may change from one group to another, but under most conditions an ectomorph is unlikely to become as muscular as the most muscular mesomorphs or as obese as the most obese endomorphs. Similarly, the most slender endomorphs are unlikely to become as slender as the most slender ectomorphs. These differences in body type appear to reflect differences in genetic traits and the responses of different types of bodies to their environments. At present, our society favors the ectomorphic

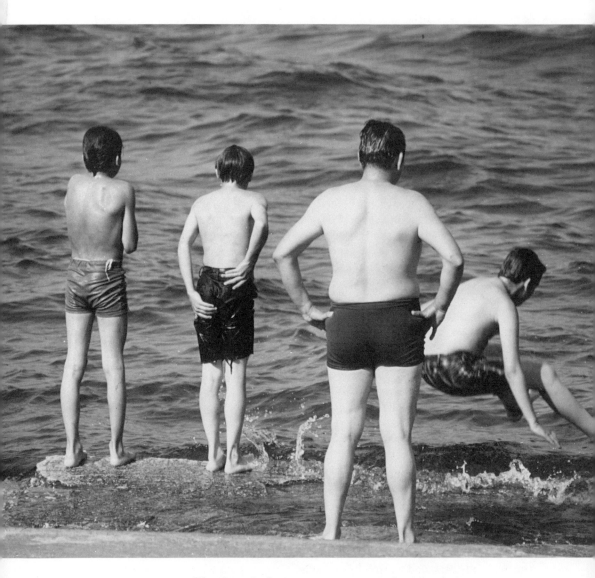

*The three body types are ectomorphs (slender),
mesomorphs (muscular), and endomorphs (obese).*

and mesomorphic body types. But endomorphs may be more efficient in their use of foods. If food becomes scarce, nature may well favor endomorphs. We should probably all follow the old adage, "Moderation in all things." As we have seen, different kinds of problems are associated with having too much or too little body fat.

Finally, the body changes form with age. As infants, the masses of the skeleton and of the muscles are relatively low, compared to the masses of these structures in adults. Between the ages of three and six months, there is an increase in the number of *adipocytes*, or fat cells, in the body. As the muscles and skeleton develop throughout childhood, the number of fat cells in the body increases, although this increase is quite slow. Adolescence brings about a rapid acceleration in skeletal and muscular development, and the number of fat cells may also increase rapidly. In general, body weight increases gradually throughout adult life until about age forty-five for males and age fifty-five for females. The increase in adult body weight may or may not involve an increase in the proportion of fat in the body. After age forty-five (males) or fifty-five (females), body weight tends to decline. Since most of the decrease results from a reduction in muscle and skeleton weight, there is usually a greater proportion of fat in the bodies of older people than there is in younger people of the same weight. Late in life, a loss of body fat contributes to the overall loss of weight. Although the evidence suggests that lean people outlive obese people, many obese people live to be quite old. It may be that people who were relatively obese all of their lives tend to live longer than those who became obese in middle age. This observation suggests that people who are "naturally" obese are better adapted to high levels of body fat than are people whose obesity results from a change in habits or diet.

Chapter Twelve

SUMMARY

As living organisms, we are completely dependent on our environment for the resources needed to remain living and healthy. We use a very wide variety of foods as sources of energy and materials. Because our requirements for many substances (for example, most of the vitamins) are modest, we are likely to meet those requirements if our diets are reasonably varied. It is not necessary that all the materials we require be present in every meal. As we have seen, we can endure considerable periods without food of any kind with little threat to our health. We can also endure short periods with poor diets, but prolonged consumption of diets lacking in proteins, vitamins, or some salts may reduce our health and shorten our lives. Similarly, excesses of some materials in our diets may also cause problems: excesses of salts, vitamins, proteins, sugars, some fats, and calories can reduce health.

It is also important to recognize that although we all share certain common requirements and limitations in the nature of our diets, individuals differ. Some of us have a limited tolerance for carbohydrates, for fats, for phenylalanine, for salts, or for a wide variety of other materials in the diet. Some of us are efficient and gain weight easily; others, perhaps less efficient, maintain a constant weight easily. For all of us, dietary requirements change as we age.

We have ignored completely the fact that some people are allergic to some foods. Obviously, this can present difficulties if such foods are major sources of required compounds. And behavior can have a powerful effect upon our nutritional state, based in part on our perception of ourselves and our response to the many aspects of our environment. Behavior also plays a role in normal nutrition. Generally, animals and humans given adequate choice will select diets that meet their needs. It is not clear how they know to do this. However, this book gives you some idea of the involvement of every part of our bodies, and of the importance of everything from our thoughts to our biochemistry, in the maintenance of good nutrition and in avoiding nutritional diseases.

Glossary

Adenosine triphosphate (ATP): A chemical compound that serves as a "chemical currency" for the storage and transfer of energy in many living organisms. When other chemicals are used as a source of energy in the body, that energy is first stored as ATP; when the body uses energy as, for example, in muscular activity, ATP is the immediate source of that energy.

Adipocytes: Fat-storage cells. Fatty tissue consists of masses of adipocytes.

Aldosterone: A hormone derived from cholesterol and produced in part of the adrenal gland, a gland located near the kidney. Aldosterone is important in regulating the salt and water content of the body through its actions in the kidney.

Amino acids: There are about twenty different amino acids, but they all contain carbon, hydrogen, oxygen and nitrogen and have a common chemical structure. Chains of amino acids are linked together to form proteins, which serve as enzymes and as structural elements in the body.

Anorectic: A person who suffers from anorexia.

Anorexia nervosa: Anorexia is the loss of appetite for food, and the term *nervosa* means that it is for emotional reasons.

Antidiuretic hormone (ADH): Also called *vasopressin,* this hormone is produced in the pituitary gland and acts upon the kidney tubule to increase its ability to take up water from the fluid that will become urine.

Atheroma: A mass which is formed when the intima (innermost layer of tissue in an artery) degenerates, thickens, and hardens, as occurs in artherosclerosis.

Biochemistry: The study of the chemical processes involved in plant and animal life.

Bulimia: An abnormal and constant craving for food.

Bulimic: A person who suffers from bulimia.

Calorie: A measure of heat. Specifically, one calorie is the amount of heat that will raise the temperature of 1 gram of water by one degree centigrade.

Cholesterol: A fat and an alcohol. It is important because it is the basis of the major male and female sex hormones and of some of the hormones that regulate the metabolism and transport of glucose. Excessively high levels in the blood seem to be associated with atherosclerosis.

Coenzymes: Organic molecules which usually contain phosphates and some vitamins. A coenzyme must unite with another protein (called an apoenzyme) in order to function as an enzyme.

Co-ion: When salts dissolve in water, at least two particles are produced, one having a positive (+) charge and the other a negative (−) charge. These charged particles are ions, and each is the co-ion for the other. Co-ions, therefore, are the oppositely charged particles that result from dissolving a salt.

(86)

Collagen: The major structural protein in the bodies of most animals. It forms the network that holds most of the organs of the body together, and our tendons and ligaments are made of collagen.

Coronary: An obstruction of the blood vessels that supply the heart muscle with blood. The word coronary refers to encirclement in the manner of a crown.

Cortisol: The main hormone produced by the adrenal glands which promotes the production of glycogen in the liver and raises the level of glucose in the blood. It also has anti-inflammatory properties and is often injected into parts of the body to reduce inflammation and the pain that results from it.

Cushing's disease: A disease characterized by obesity, especially of the head, neck and trunk, the appearance of brownish streaks on the abdominal wall, muscular weakness, and the development of weak, porous bones. It appears to be the result of malfunctions of either the pituitary or of part of the adrenal glands.

Diabetes insipidus: A form of diabetes (water loss through urination) that is the result of an inherited defect in the kidney tubules.

Diabetes mellitus: This form of diabetes is a result of the high sugar (glucose) content of the blood which, in turn, is a result of the failure of the pancreas to produce insulin.

Edema: A condition in which there is an abnormal accumulation of fluid in the intercellular spaces of the body, giving the body (usually the legs and feet) a soft, puffy appearance.

Enzymes: Substances which catalyze (speed up) reactions between other chemicals but which remain unchanged by such reactions. Enzymes are proteins and they may be combined with either fat or sugars.

Epithelia: The layers of cells that cover both the external and internal parts of the body. The surface of your skin and the lining of your mouth are examples of epithelia.

Estrogens: The female sex hormones. They are derived from cholesterol.

Fatty acids: Molecules that consist of a long chain of carbon and hydrogen atoms linked together, with a carbon and two oxygens linked together at one end to form what chemists call an "acid" group. They are one of the forms in which fats are stored and transported within the body.

Fibrin: The protein that forms a blood clot.

Fibrinogen: One of several proteins important in the process of blood clotting. It is converted to fibrin in the presence of thrombin.

Glucagon: A hormone produced in the pancreas. One of its major actions is to cause cells in the liver to break down glycogen into the sugar glucose, and to release the glucose into the blood. Glucagon and insulin act as a team: glucagon increases the amount of glucose in the blood and insulin decreases it.

Hypothalamus: Part of the base of the brain and an important site for the coordination of the functions of the endocrine and nervous system. The pituitary gland is suspended from the base of the hypothalamus and receives many of its signals from it.

Insulin: A protein produced by cells in the pancreas. It serves as a hormone; that is, it is produced in one part of the body, released into the blood, and has its actions in another part of the body. Among its many actions, insulin causes cells, particularly fat cells and muscle cells, to take up sugar (glucose) from the blood. It is produced in inadequate amounts by people who have sugar diabetes.

Kilocalorie: This unit is simply equal to one thousand calories; that is, it is the amount of heat that will raise 1,000 grams (one kilogram) of water by one degree centigrade. It is sometimes written as "Calorie," and the capital "C" indicates that it is really a kilocalorie. This is the Calorie we are familiar with as a measure of the energy content of foods. If a food has 20 Calories per ounce, it means that, if the food were burned, an amount of heat equal to 20 kilocalories would be released. The same amount of heat is released when the food is used in the body, but, of course, at a lower temperature.

Kwashiorkor: A disease caused by lack of protein in the diet.

Malnutrition: A condition in which the diet provides enough calories to sustain life, but lacks essential ingredients, such as certain vitamins or proteins.

Metabolism: The sum of all the physical and chemical processes by which living material is produced and maintained. It also includes the chemical reactions by which energy is made available for use by organisms and, therefore, can be measured in units of heat (kilocalories).

Osmosis: The flow of water from a region in which it (the water) is in highest concentration to a region in which it is in lowest concentration.

Osteomalacia: A disease in which the bones become soft due to a reduction in their mineral content, particularly of calcium. It is usually a result of deficiencies in vitamin D.

Osteoporosis: A disease in which the bones become thinner and more fragile. It tends to be associated with advancing age and it is more common and more serious in women than in men.

Pancreas: A gland located near the stomach. One part of it releases enzymes into the intestine where they break down food, and other parts of the gland produce the hormones insulin and glucagon, which are released into the blood.

Parathyroid glands: Four small glands located near (*para-*) the thyroid gland in the neck. They produce a hormone called *parathyroid hormone*, important for the regulation of the levels of calcium in the blood and for bone production.

Phenylalanine hydroxylase: An enzyme that converts the amino acid phenylalanine to tyrosine. It is absent or deficient in persons with phenylketonuria (PKU), and it is important for growth in infants and for nitrogen metabolism in adults.

Physiology: The study of how living organisms function.

(89)

Pituitary gland: The gland located just below the brain and above the nose and mouth, it has major importance as a site of communication between the nervous system and the several glands that secrete their hormones into the blood. Together, all of these glands are referred to as the endocrine system.

Platelets: Disk-shaped structures in the blood of all mammals. They have an important role in the clotting mechanism of blood and become activated by the presence of thrombin.

Prothrombin: A protein found in normal blood plasma. It is converted to thrombin by prothrombin activator.

Rebound deficiency: A condition that often develops when a person has taken large amounts of a drug or vitamin for a long time and then stops or reduces the amount suddenly. Under these conditions, the body may behave as though there were a deficiency of the drug or vitamin, even if the person continues to take a dose that would normally be adequate.

Receptor cells: The part of the sensory nervous system that first detects a signal in the environment (light, odors, etc.) and converts it into an electrical signal in the nervous system.

Rhodopsin: A light-sensitive protein that has a purple-red color when it has been kept in the dark and which bleaches to a yellow color in the light. It is an important part of the sensory cells in our eyes because it absorbs light and starts the processes that result in our ability to see light. It is derived from vitamin A.

Sclerosis: A general term for any hardening of normally soft tissues in the body, especially for those due to inflammation. When it occurs in the arteries, it is called arteriosclerosis.

Sensible: Refers to those losses of weight that can be "sensed" as, for example, urination, fecal losses, and the loss of water as perspiration. *Insensible* refers to those losses of weight that cannot be "sensed." These include losses of water through the skin that are not apparent perspiration, losses of water in exhaled air, and losses of body weight as carbon dioxide in exhaled air.

Thrombin: A protein that converts another protein, called fibrinogen (Factor I) to fibrin.

Sensory system: That part of the nervous system that is involved with sensation: for example, our capacities for touch, vision, and hearing are due to the operation of the sensory system.

Sympathetic nervous system: A part of the nervous system called the autonomic nervous system is involved with the maintenance of functions we never think about, such as blood pressure, body temperature, etc. The sympathetic nervous system is that part of the autonomic system that tends to speed things up or to prepare the body for action, as in a fight with a rival or an escape from a predator.

Triglycerides: Fats made from a compound known as *glycerin* linked to three fatty acids. They are an important form of fats for storage and, in a slightly modified form, are found commonly in the membranes of cells.

Undernutrition: A condition in which the diet includes all of the basic dietary requirements, but is less than the minimum amount of food required for maintenance of a constant weight.

For Further Reading

Adler, Irving. *Food*. New York: John Day, 1977.

Baldwin, Dorothy, and Lister, Claire. *Your Body Fuel*. New York: The Bookwright Press, 1984.

Coles, Robert. *Still Hungry in America*. New York: World Publishing Co., 1969

Eagles, Douglas A. *Your Weight*. New York: Franklin Watts, 1982.

Franz, Barbara E., and Franz, William S. *Nutritional Survival Manual for the 80's: A Young People's Guide to Dietary Goals for the United States*. New York: Julian Messner, 1981.

Gilbert, Sara. *You Are What You Eat*. New York: Macmillan Publishing Co., Inc., 1977.

Jones, Hettie. *How to Eat Your ABC's: A Book About Vitamins*. New York: Four Winds Press, 1976.

Landau, Elaine. *Why are They Starving Themselves?: Understanding Anorexia Nervosa and Bulimia*. New York: Julian Messner, 1983.

Matthews, Dee. *The You Can Do It! Kids Diet*. New York: Holt, Rinehart & Winston, 1985.

Peavy, Linda, and Smith, Ursula. *Food, Nutrition and You*. New York: Charles Scribner's Sons, 1982.

Riedman, Sarah R. *Diabetes*. New York: Franklin Watts, 1980.

Seixas, Judith S. *Junk Food—What It Is, What It Does*. New York: Greenwillow Books, 1984.

Seixas, Judith S. *Vitamins—What They Are, What They Do*. New York: Greenwillow Books, 1986.

White, Marlene B., and White, William C. Jr. *Bulimarexia: The Binge-Purge Cycle*. New York: Norton, 1983.

Index